FIFTY PLACES TO BIKE
BEFORE YOU DIE

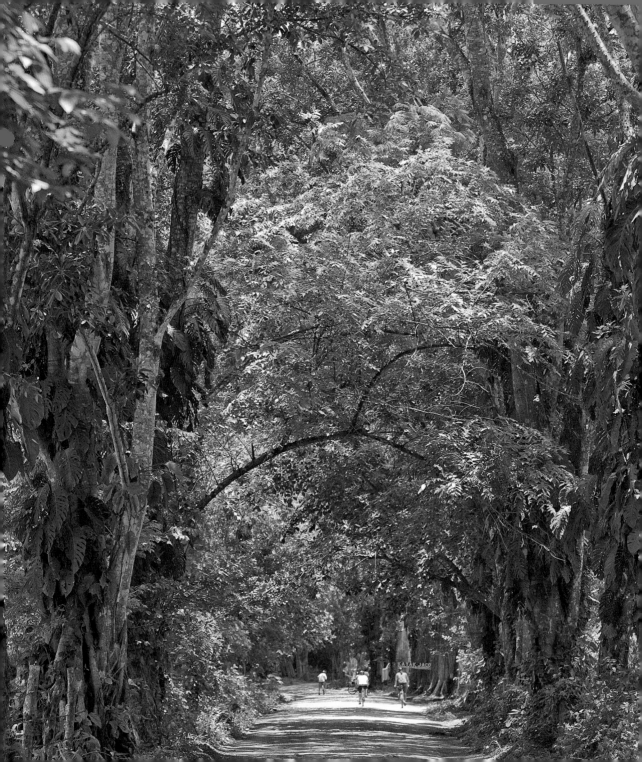

FIFTY PLACES TO
BIKE
BEFORE YOU DIE

Biking Experts Share the World's Greatest Destinations

Chris Santella

FOREWORD BY JOE "METAL COWBOY" KURMASKIE

ABRAMS IMAGE

NEW YORK

This book is for my girls, Cassidy, Annabel, and Deidre.
I hope many more miles await us on our bikes.

Fifty More Places to Fly Fish Before You Die:
Fly-Fishing Experts Share More of the World's Greatest Destinations

Fifty Places to Fly Fish Before You Die:
Fly-Fishing Experts Share the World's Greatest Destinations

Fifty Places to Play Golf Before You Die:
Golf Experts Share the World's Greatest Destinations

Fifty Favorite Fly-Fishing Tales:
Expert Fly Anglers Share Stories from the Sea and Stream

Fifty Places to Sail Before You Die:
Sailing Experts Share the World's Greatest Destinations

Fifty Places to Go Birding Before You Die:
Birding Experts Share the World's Greatest Destinations

Fifty Places to Dive Before You Die:
Diving Experts Share the World's Greatest Destinations

Fifty Places to Hike Before You Die:
Outdoor Experts Share the World's Greatest Destinations

Once in a Lifetime Trips:
The World's Fifty Most Extraordinary and Memorable Travel Experiences

Fifty More Places to Play Golf Before You Die:
Golf Experts Share the World's Greatest Destinations

Contents

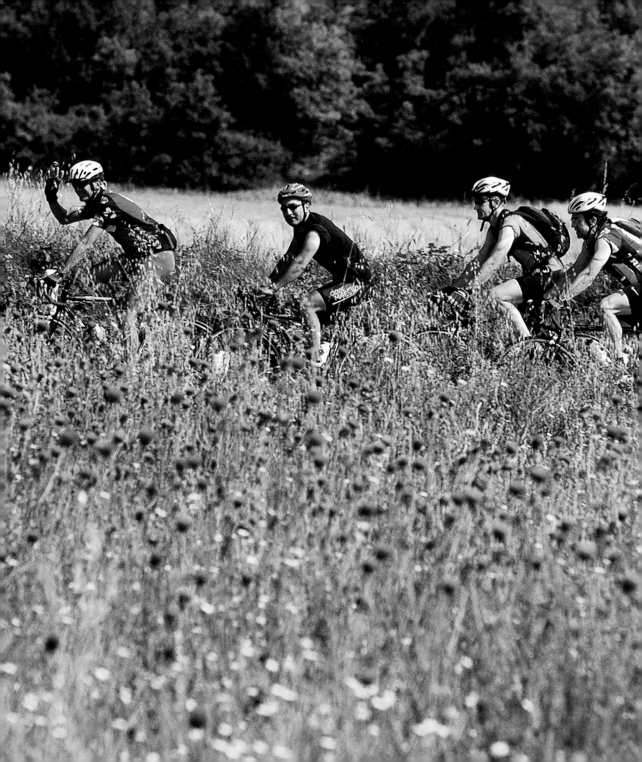

ACKNOWLEDGMENTS

This book would not have been possible without the generous assistance of the expert cyclists who shared their time and experience to help bring these fifty great bicycling venues to life. To these men and women, I offer the most heartfelt thanks. I also wish to acknowledge the fine efforts of my agent, Stephanie Kip Rostan; my editors, Wesley Royce and Jennifer Levesque; designer Anna Christian; and copyeditor Ashley Benning, who all helped bring the book into being. Finally, I want to extend a special thanks to my wife, Deidre, and my daughters Cassidy and Annabel, who've humored my absence during seemingly endless deadlines, and to my parents, Tina and Andy Santella, who are not cyclists, but always encouraged me to pursue my passions.

FOREWORD

There's a revolutionary living under your roof. It doesn't chant slogans or engage in armed resistance, but it's a power to be reckoned with all the same. It bunks down in the garage, hangs from the rafters, or waits patiently by the door. To some it's disguised as a child's toy, a deceptively simple device for recreating on the weekends. In truth, bikes are lightning strikes in a top tube; a rebel with a cause just waiting to invigorate your life; Gandhi, Malcolm X, and The Clash in motion rolling down the road on some madcap adventure of freedom and discovery. They're Teddy Roosevelt and all of his damn Rough Riders running roughshod over sloth, the ordinary, and sedentary living. They're a symphony one day and an all-night rave the next. Pedal a bike and you'll have all the proof you need of a balanced universe. The bicycle has saved drunks, junkies, and quietly discontented accountants alike. It's defibbed couch potatoes out of the coma of the mushy twilight of a TV's glow, and it's turned back time for retirees who thought their best days were done. Quite simply, the bicycle is a time machine taking everyone who climbs on back to a ten-year-old self who believed in speed and the gorgeous savage inside. But like all time machines, it's not just the when of the matter that's important, but also the where. You'll have an "experience" no matter where you roll, since the bicycle makes you a traveler rather than a tourist, but there's something to be said for hedging your bets. That's where *Fifty Places to Bike Before You Die* takes over as a road map to peak experiences in the saddle. From pedaling wine country to rolling up to the largest baobab in the African bush, why to go where and when have been distilled for you. All that's left is to point your wheels, find your rhythm, and go as long and far as your desire will take you.

—JOE "METAL COWBOY" KURMASKIE

INTRODUCTION

There are faster ways to get from point A to B than by bicycle. But as anyone who's spent any time on a bike knows, there are few more pleasurable ways to really appreciate a place . . . while raising your heart rate!

I wrote *Fifty Places to Bike Before You Die* for those who value life in the slower lane, and the chance to make a closer connection to people and places along the open road.

"What makes a destination a place you have to bike before you die?" you might ask. The chance to take in sweeping mountain or coastal scenery? To sample fine wines and cuisine (with a little less guilt, as you'll be riding the calories off)? The promise of interaction with people in remote places, whose cultures have changed little over hundreds of years? The answer would be yes to all of the above, and an abundance of other criteria. One thing I knew when I began this project—I was *NOT* the person to assemble this list. So I followed a recipe that served me well in my first eight *Fifty Places* books—to seek the advice of some professionals. To write *Fifty Places to Bike Before You Die*, I interviewed a host of people closely connected with the cycling world and asked them to share some of their favorite experiences. These experts range from well-known tour leaders (like Dan Austin, George Butterfield, and Lauren Hefferon) to equipment manufacturers (like Paul McKenzie) and journalists (like Joe Kurmaskie and Joe Parkin). Some spoke of venues that are near and dear to their hearts, places where they've built their professional reputations; others spoke of places they've only visited once, but that made a profound impression. People appreciate biking for many different reasons, and this range of attractions is evidenced here. (To give a sense of the breadth of the interviewees' outdoor backgrounds, a bio of each individual is included after each essay.)

Biking means different things to different people. For some, it may mean grinding out 75 or 100 miles a day on a mountainous road, barely pausing to gobble an energy bar and down some water; for others, it may be a means to the end of tasting fine Pinot Noirs. *Fifty Places to Bike Before You Die* attempts to capture the spectrum of biking experiences. While the book collects fifty great biking experiences, it by no means attempts to rank the places discussed, or the quality of the experiences afforded there. Such ranking is, of course, largely subjective: The appeals of riding 310 miles without

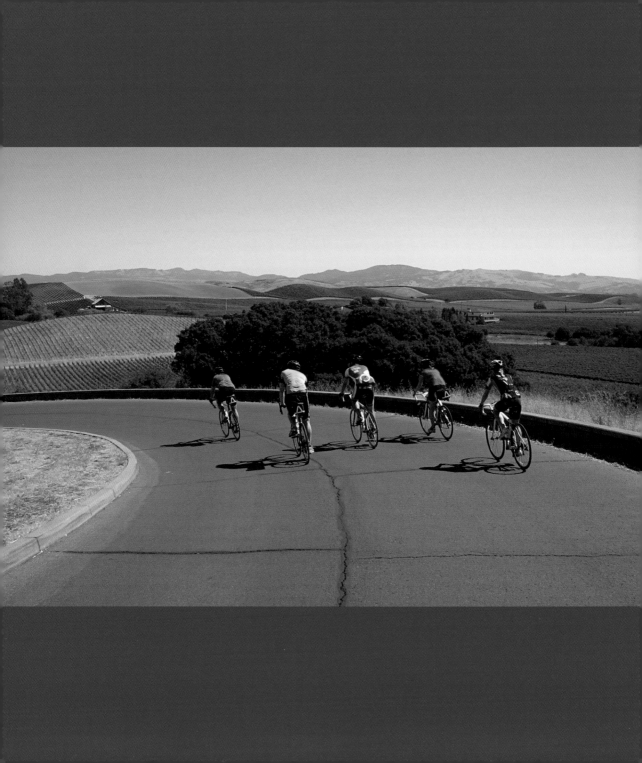

stopping may be anathema to someone who's more interested in a casual inn-to-inn ride in France, or merely commuting to work in Portland, Oregon.

In the hope that a few readers might embark on their own adventures, I have provided brief "If You Go" information at the end of each chapter, including the names of outfitters who offer supported rides in the region at hand (if applicable). The "If You Go" information is by no means a comprehensive list, but should give would-be travelers a starting point for planning their trip. (Please note: The "If You Go" information includes an entry for "Level of Difficulty." This assumes the individual is riding the entire course of the route described. Supported rides—that is, rides with a van that carries your bags—can generally give riders a little help on longer or steeper days. Likewise, rides that are classified as "easy" or "intermediate" can often be supplemented with extra miles to increase their challenge.)

One needn't travel to the ends of the earth to find a rewarding biking experience. Yet a trip to a dream venue can create memories for a lifetime. It's my hope that this little book will inspire you to embark on some new biking adventures of your own.

—CHRIS SANTELLA

OPPOSITE:
New vintages await around every bend in California's Wine Country.
NEXT PAGE:
Bicycle tourists are just beginning to discover the possibilities of Bali.

13

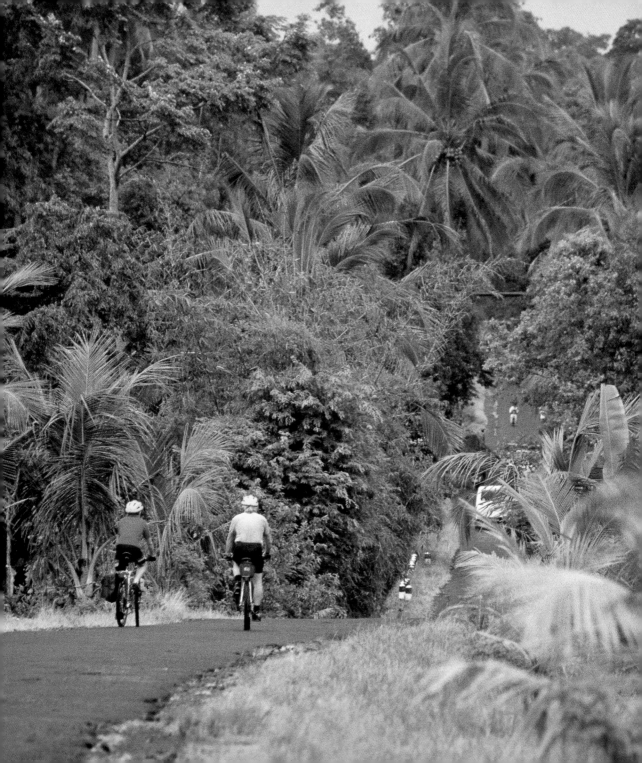

The Destinations

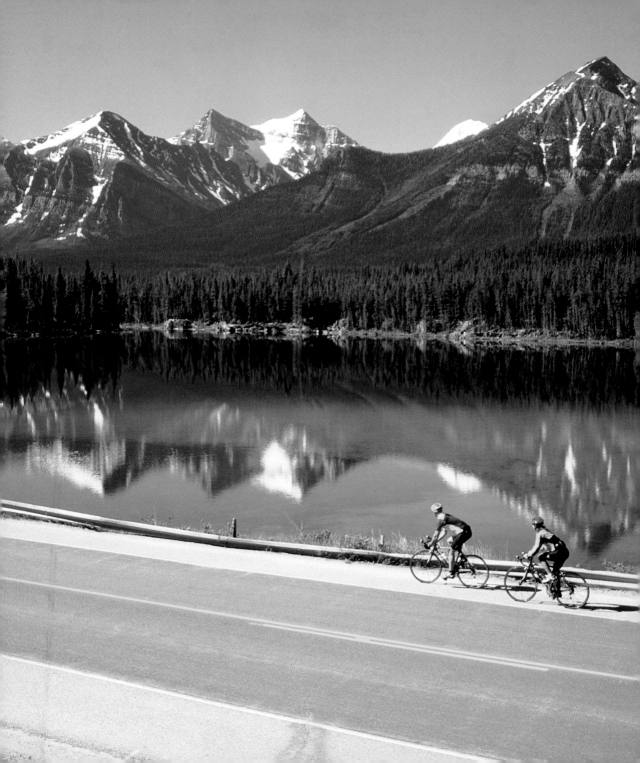

THE ICEFIELDS PARKWAY

RECOMMENDED BY **Peter Weiland**

Simply put—Alberta's Icefields Parkway may be the most accessible and most beautiful mountain road in the world. It certainly changed Peter Weiland's life. "I came to Canada from Germany as a student and did a ride from Calgary to Banff to Jasper, then on to the coast of British Columbia. The ride through Jasper touched me in so many ways. It was the catalyst for me to immigrate to Canada and start my career leading bike tours.

"There are so many aspects of the ride that set it apart. First, you're cycling through two national parks and UNESCO World Heritage sites—Jasper and Banff—and you're entirely in those parks, landscapes that are nearly untouched by humans beyond the road. You get a real sense of being immersed in a mountain wilderness as you parallel the Continental Divide, from the one hundred glaciers in view from the road to the bear, elk, moose, caribou, bighorn sheep—even wolves—you might see. There are several memorable lodges—not opulent, but places that really give you a sense of place and of an earlier time. And there are several short but very memorable hikes you can do when you're not in the saddle. I've ridden the Icefields Parkway in one day—142 miles (230 km). But I would recommend that visitors do it in a more leisurely five days."

Peter recommends that you ride north to south. "The north faces of the mountains have the glaciers; hence the scenery is more spectacular if you're riding toward them," he advised. After shuttling from Calgary to the town of Jasper (about a six-hour drive), you'll have an afternoon to linger at Lac Beauvert or tune up your bike (you won't see another bike shop for 100-plus miles!) before setting out on the ride the following day. Your first day in the saddle starts out gently, following the Athabasca River out of Jasper. Not far along, Peter likes to detour from the main Icefields Parkway onto the Old Icefields Parkway. "It's a little bumpy, but very lightly traveled by cars," he said. "Since it's so quiet,

OPPOSITE:
There are few
(if any) more
spectacular
mountain rides
than the Icefields
Parkway.

there's a good opportunity to view wildlife. This road leads us to Mt. Edith Cavell and Angel Glacier. You have the option to bike up to the viewing point—an 1,800-foot climb over 8 miles (13 km) (I like to think of it as the 'Mont Ventoux' climb of the Canadian Rockies)—or to shuttle up. At the top, you're treated to the sight of the glacier, hanging below a vertical mountain face and above a lake where icebergs (calved from the glacier) float. Those who opt to ride to the top are rewarded with a great switchback descent."

Day two takes you along the Sunwapta River valley (another fertile stretch for wildlife sightings) and on to the Columbia Icefields—headwaters of the Athabasca, North Saskatchewan, and Columbia Rivers; it's the largest ice field south of the Arctic Circle. "Much of this day's ride (32 miles [51 km] in total) climbs gently along the Sunwapta, though at the end, it's 12 percent grade," Peter continued. "The views are amazing as you climb, though; you have many good excuses to get off your bike and snap photos. We stop for the day across from the Athabasca Glacier at Icefields Inn. That afternoon, we take a short hike up to Parker Ridge, considered one of the best short hikes in the Canadian Rockies. At the top, you're rewarded with a bird's-eye view of Saskatchewan Glacier."

Day three is the longest day on the Icefields Parkway and takes you to the highest point on any paved road in Canada . . . if you so desire. But it's not all uphill. "After a gentle climb to Sunwapta Pass, you have the longest descent of the ride, roughly 10 miles (16 km) down to the Weeping Wall on the Saskatchewan River, a deep canyon face with many waterfalls trickling out," Peter described. "The next 31 miles (50 km) follow the Saskatchewan River. It's fairly flat, and the miles fly by. The afternoon will be spent climbing the 20 miles (32 km) to Bow Pass. It's not all uphill, but there are two good climbs. I like to call the Bow Pass region 'the lake district.' Lower and Upper Waterfall Lake are a lovely turquoise, and they're surrounded by big mountain spires. There's the option to ride to the summit to view Peyto Lake, called the bluest lake in the Canadian Rockies. If you're not in need of an oxygen tent, it'll be only seven or eight minutes to get to the top—7,000 feet. From here it's just another 5 miles (8 km) to Bow Lake, Bow Glacier, and Num-ti-jah Lodge. This lodge takes you back in time. The first section was built in 1940, the remainder completed in 1950. Your stay is capped off with a spectacular dinner in the Elkhorn Dining Room. Buffalo and elk steaks, caribou medallions, and other game are featured on the menu. After dinner, we usually fire up the old sauna that was built in the woods next to the lodge. You heat up in the sauna and then jump into Bow Lake. After a few rotations between the sauna and the lake, you feel like a newborn.

There's nothing like accomplishing a great ride and then topping it off with a historic sauna experience."

Day four brings you back to the relative civilization of Lake Louise. The Icefields Parkway officially ends here, and the Trans-Canada Highway takes over. "We like to go up to Lake Louise," Peter continued, "and there's an option to ride up the old tram line. It's a crushed gravel bike path, but there's no car exhaust. If you have a lot of energy left, you can hike up to the teahouse at Lake Agness or do the famous Plain of Six Glaciers hike. On the final day, we take the Bow Valley Parkway into Banff, which is 40 miles (64 km) southeast along the Bow River. Most cars take the Trans-Canada, so we have the road mostly to ourselves."

PETER WEILAND took over Rocky Mountain Cycle Tours in 1999. His deep love for big mountains and wild places brought him to Canada from Germany. Peter is very passionate about all aspects of cycling and has pioneered several amazing road and mountain bike tours in the Canadian West and on the island of Majorca, Spain. In the winter he works as a ski guide at Whistler Blackcomb. He lives with his wife and three kids in British Columbia.

If You Go

▶ **Getting There:** Calgary is served by many major carriers, including Air Canada (888-247-2262; www.aircanada.com).

▶ **Best Time to Visit:** Roads are generally clear of snow late June until late September.

▶ **Guides/Outfitters:** Companies that lead tours on the Icefields Parkway include Rocky Mountain Cycle (800-661-2453; www.rockymountaincycle.com).

▶ **Level of Difficulty:** The tour described here is 190 miles (300 km) over five riding days. It's rated moderate to difficult.

▶ **Accommodations:** There are lodging options in Jasper and Banff. In between, Peter likes the following spots: Sunwapta Falls Resort (888-828-5777; sunwapta.com), Glacier View Inn (866-875-8456; www.nationalparkreservations.com), Num-ti-jah Lodge (403-522-2167; sntj.ca), and Deer Lodge (403-522-3991; www.crmr.com/deer).

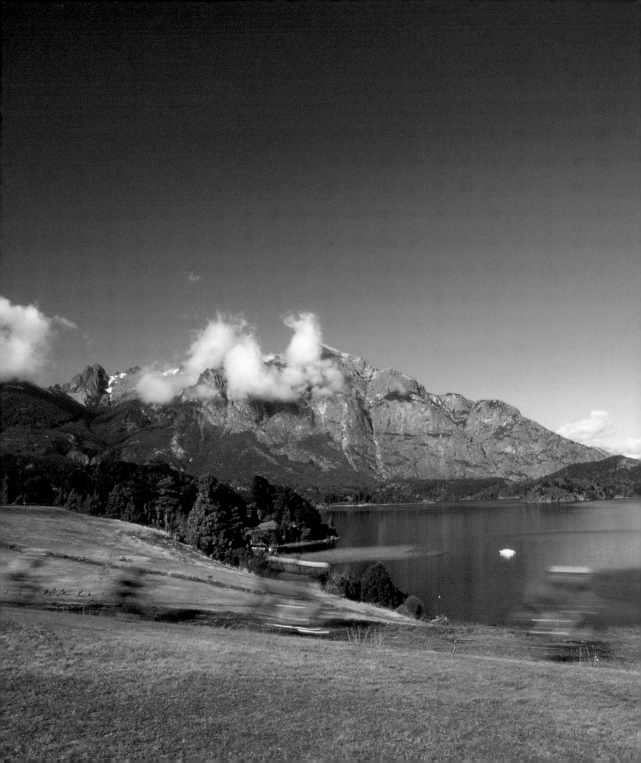

SEVEN LAKES DISTRICT

RECOMMENDED BY **Adam Ballard**

"I didn't come to Argentine Patagonia with too many expectations," Adam Ballard began. "I imagined that I'd be cycling in some beautiful alpine settings, among lakes, mountains, and villages reminiscent of ski towns in Switzerland. My aesthetic hopes were certainly met and then some; the Seven Lakes region is sublimely beautiful. What surprised me was how much of a biking culture—especially mountain biking—there was in Argentina. You encounter many Argentines out on the trails or road, and the bicycling connects you. The Seven Lakes District between Bariloche and San Martín de los Andes is becoming the outdoor adventure capital of Argentina. You might compare the towns to Jackson Hole—developed toward higher-end visitors, but still near wilderness. The food culture—especially the *asado*—also struck me as wonderful and unique."

Similar to Texas, Patagonia is as much a state of mind as a place. Encompassing roughly 400,000 square miles of infinite steppes, groaning glaciers, spiky pink granite peaks, and electric-blue lakes, wind-pummeled Patagonia is still very much a frontier. While it is relatively easy to disappear for weeks on end into one of the region's vast national parks, an expanding infrastructure of facilities for ecotourists seeking lodging beyond a tent or hostel makes it equally possible to travel quite comfortably.

The Lake District of Argentina rests in the northern section of Patagonia, in the provinces of Río Negro and Neuquén, and like Patagonia itself extends across the Andes to the west into Chile. For most bicyclists, the region is demarcated by Bariloche in the south and San Martín de los Andes in the north; many itineraries travel between the two towns.

"I began my trip just outside of Bariloche at Llao Llao, a wonderful property in a spectacular setting in Nahuel Huapi National Park, between Nahuel Huapi and Moreno Lakes," Adam continued. "Llao Llao is a national park lodge. The difference, though,

OPPOSITE:
A vista from
Seven Lakes
Road, which
is destined to
become one of
the world's
greatest rides.

between it and the Old Faithful Inn in Yellowstone is that this inn is incredibly well-appointed. It's considered one of the finest hotel properties in Argentina. There's one fantastic ride that embarks right from the lodge. You cycle down to a small landing on Lake Nahuel Huapi, and then take a boat across it to the Quetrihué Peninsula in Los Arrayanes National Park. The scenery is tremendous; there are mountain spires shooting up on either side and forested peninsulas extending into the lake. The trail in the national park runs through a forest of gorgeous arrayáns—the namesake for the park. These trees have an incredibly red bark, somewhat reminiscent of the madrones you might find along the west coast of the United States. Though it's a single-track trail, it's quite doable for beginning mountain bikers. I have to count this as one of the most pristine rides I've ever done."

For cyclists seeking a challenge, one ride stands out—Ruta de los Siete Lagos, or Seven Lakes Road. The road traverses the Andes from the village of La Angostura (near Los Arrayanes) north to San Martín de los Andes, some 70 miles (112 km) away. (There are actually eight lakes along the road—Nahuel Huapi, Espejo, Correntoso, Escondido, Villarino, Falkner, Machónico, and Lácar as you head from south to north.) It can be done in a day, though many will stretch the ride out over several days (there are campgrounds and modest *hosterias* along the way) to drink in the scenery and enjoy the lakes. "The road cuts into the heart of the mountains in Parque Nacional Nahuel Huapi," Adam added, "and there are really no towns or settlements en route. Here, the road is the thing. Part of the road is still unpaved, though that project is under way. When the work is complete, it will no doubt be one of the all-time great road routes in the world.

"The ride starts in a forested mountain setting, with a great deal of up and down. As you climb through the closed mountain valleys, the views begin to open up. Vistas get bigger and broader as you reach the halfway point, and the area takes on a high desert quality, not unlike the canyons of the southwestern United States. I remember reaching a high point on the road above one of the brilliant blue lakes with snowcapped peaks all around, with a smile stretching ear to ear. I felt like I was on top of the world. Things get even better toward the end of the ride. You're about 10.5 miles (17 km) above the town of San Martín de los Andes—from this point, it's all downhill. If you've done the ride in a day, you've worked pretty hard, but you get this great reward. The road is paved here, and you bomb down the hill into this lovely resort town. The ride into town is so fun, I did the climb back up the following day for the thrill of cruising down again."

As alluded to above, no trip to Argentine Patagonia is complete without attending at least one *asado* . . . even if you don't partake of meat. "It's a quintessential part of the Argentine experience," Adam said. "An *asado* can feature a host of roasted and grilled meats, and perhaps some vegetables too. The most traditional *asado* features a lamb splayed open and roasted over an open wood fire. The meat's incredibly tender, with a wood smoke flavor—some of the best lamb you'll ever eat. As an appetizer, I also sampled *provoleta*, which is grilled provolone cheese, seasoned with herbs. It reaches a potential that you wouldn't expect. All gets washed down with an assortment of local Malbecs, and a white varietal called Torrontes, which is becoming quite popular in Argentina."

A DAM B ALLARD has been guiding bicycle tours for Backroads since 2008. He's led trips in Yellowstone, Martha's Vineyard, California, Costa Rica and Peru, Argentina and Patagonia. Before joining Backroads, Adam worked as the acquisitions specialist and reclassification implementation coordinator with Robert Crown Law Library at Stanford University. He is a graduate of Dartmouth College, where he majored in music.

If You Go

▶ **Getting There:** The trip begins and ends in Bariloche, which is served from Buenos Aires by Aerolineas Argentinas (800-333-0276; www.aerolineas.com.ar) and LAN (866-435-9526; www.lan.com).

▶ **Best Time to Visit:** The austral spring and summer—October through March.

▶ **Guides/Outfitters:** Several outfitters conduct biking excursions in the Seven Lakes District, including Backroads (800-462-2848; www.backroads.com).

▶ **Level of Difficulty:** The itinerary described above entails seven days of riding, some on dirt and single-track. Distances are generally not great, but difficulty is rated moderate to challenging.

▶ **Accommodations:** The Backroads itinerary includes stays at several higher-end properties, including Llao Llao (+54 2944 448 530; www.llaollao.com), Las Balsas (+54 2944 494 308; www.lasbalsas.com), and Antares Patagonia Suites (+54 2972 427 670; www .antarespatagonia-sma.com). Camping and other more modest accommodations are available at several points along the Seven Lakes Road.

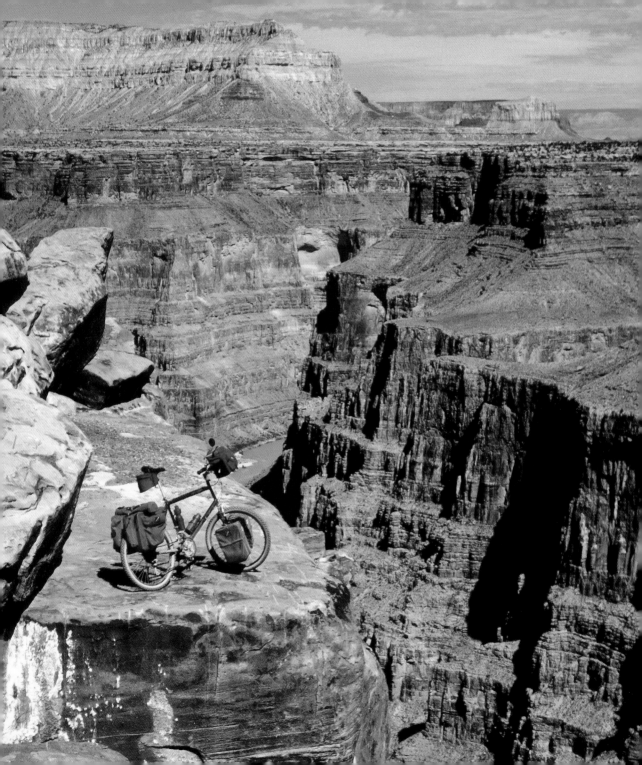

GRAND CANYON—NORTH RIM

RECOMMENDED BY **Jared Fisher**

Few if any visitors come away from the Grand Canyon unmoved—whether one steps off a tour bus and peers over the edge of the South Rim for thirty minutes or traverses the canyon from north to south. For Jared Fisher, the best way to experience the wonders of one of the planet's most awe-inspiring erosion events is to bike upon the Kaibab Plateau, high above the canyon's North Rim.

"There are several factors that make the Kaibab Plateau a very special place to ride," he elaborated. "First, the plateau is not very hilly. It's pretty mellow for a mountain biking tour, a great trip to introduce 'roadies' to cycling in the dirt. It's really like a rolling meadow.

"People usually associate the Grand Canyon with heat, but that isn't the case on the North Rim. You're 1,000 feet higher than on the South Rim, and as a result it's much cooler, plus you have very different flora; here, it's more ponderosa pines and aspens than cacti. (The elevation at some points on the Kaibab is near 9,000 feet.) The North Rim is also spared the crowds that you see at the South Rim. They get an average of four million visitors a year. On the North Rim, it's more like forty thousand. When I'm out for five days, I can generally count how many people I see on one hand—a forest ranger or two is all. From a riding perspective, it provides lots of options—folks who want a fuller day of riding have lots of choices once we get to camp. The roadies appreciate this.

"Finally, there are the spectacular views that vary each day. From the Kaibab, you get two very distinct perspectives of the canyon. When you're on the top of the plateau, you get a bird's-eye view of the canyon from 3,000 feet off the valley floor. You also can see the East Rim of the North Rim of the Grand Canyon—the site where the canyon is coming through the desert, like a train coming toward a tunnel. Seeing that cut is one of my favorite points on the trip."

OPPOSITE:

A ride on the Kaibab Plateau showcases some of the Grand Canyon's least visited wonders.

A five-day ride along the North Rim builds in momentum. The first day takes you along the old Arizona Trail, through mountain meadows and ponderosa pines. "You're riding along in the woods, a nice easy ride to acclimate to the altitude," Jared described. "Then it's like there's a cymbal crash, and suddenly you're on the East Rim. There's the drop of the Grand Canyon, but there's also that great cut, as if sliced from a giant piece of cake. People just freak out." The second day continues along the Arizona Trail, skirting along the massive plateau. (Kaibab, incidentally, means "mountain lying down" in the language of the Anasazi.) Once again, riders come through the woods to another cymbal-crashing vista. "This is the highest point on the plateau," Jared continued. "You're at the point where the Grand Canyon collides with the Kaibab. There's this feeling that as we have rolled through the woods, the canyon has snuck up and found us." The day concludes with a 5-mile hike that offers ever-shifting views of Point Imperial.

Day three takes riders down a combination of double-track trail and fire roads to North Timp Point and vistas over the main part of the canyon. "This portion of the ride—about 25 miles (40 km)—is mostly downhill," Jared said. "When you come out of the woods, you're 1,500 feet lower than where you started, low enough that there are cacti at the edge of the canyon. You're still at almost 8,000 feet, but heat rises up from the canyon to nurture the cacti. It's an odd assortment of flora. You have cacti at the rim, and 1,000 feet back, there are ponderosa pines and aspens."

The fourth day above the canyon may comprise the world's most scenic single-track ride—the Rainbow Rim Trail. "I like to describe it as if you're riding out on a series of fingers that stick out into the Grand Canyon," Jared continued. "At the knuckle of the finger, you're 2,000 feet above the canyon floor. At the fingernail, it's 5,000 feet down. All in all, you have more than twenty different viewpoints along the way. You might also come upon the Kaibab squirrel, which lives only on the plateau. They are black with a big, white bushy tail and pointy ears that look like shirt collars that are being worn up. Though it's a single track, the ride is very mellow."

On the ride's final day, you roll down the edge of the plateau to Indian Hollow, mostly on jeep roads. "We end at an elevation of 6,000 feet," Jared added. "It gets warmer as we head down—you get a sense of how hot it could've been had you been in the canyon all along, but it's only for a few hours, so it's bearable. The flora and fauna change as you descend. You definitely get a different sense of the Grand Canyon from the previous days."

Peering out from the Rainbow Rim Trail is a defining moment of a ride along the Kaibab Plateau. An even more dramatic moment comes at North Timp Point, where riders camp for nights three and four of the trip. "There's a special spot near this camp that I've been visiting for twenty years," Jared described, "a pedestal that sticks up from down the canyon wall, maybe 50 or 60 feet. There's a tiny juniper on top, maybe 2 feet tall. We call it Mr. Miyagi's House, from a scene in the movie *Karate Kid*. After dinner, once it's getting dark, we hike down the canyon with our headlamps on about 150 feet to the base of the pedestal and then climb back up. At the top, it's no bigger than a compact car. When the moon is full, you can see all the way to the bottom of the canyon. You feel like you're in your own world. If there's ever been a place to be at one with the universe or God—to have a feeling of unsurpassed peacefulness—Mr. Miyagi's House is it."

JARED FISHER founded Escape Adventures in 1992. The outfitter leads sustainable biking, hiking, and multisport tours around the Southwest, utilizing a fleet of clean-burning vegetable oil–powered support vehicles. Escape Adventures is the first fully carbon-neutral adventure outfitter in the world. Jared also owns and operates Moab Cyclery and Las Vegas Cyclery. His mountain biking, road biking, running, and hiking adventures have taken him throughout the southwestern United States and the South Pacific.

If You Go

▶ **Getting There:** Guests generally fly into Las Vegas (served by most major carriers) and take a shuttle to the ride's starting point in Fredonia, Arizona.

▶ **Best Time to Visit:** Visitors bike the North Rim from mid-spring through early fall. Thanks to its high altitude, the North Rim remains clement in the summer.

▶ **Guides/Outfitters:** There are several tour companies leading rides along the North Rim, including Escape Adventures (800-596-2953; www.escapeadventures.com).

▶ **Level of Difficulty:** The itinerary above includes five days of riding, an average of 30 miles a day. Though much of the riding is off-road, it's rated moderate.

▶ **Accommodations:** If you want to spend an extra night around the North Rim, the nearest lodging option is Grand Canyon Lodge—North Rim (877-386-4383; www.grand canyonlodgenorth.com).

DESTINATION 4

WESTERN TASMANIA

RECOMMENDED BY **Richard Oddy**

The Australian state of Tasmania rests some 150 miles (241 km) south across the Bass Strait from Melbourne; it's sometimes called "the island off the island." It's Australia but not the Australia overseas visitors imagine based on tour brochures. To put things in perspective, Tasmania is more than one-third larger than Switzerland. Although the highest peak is just above 5,000 feet, Tasmania is considered the most mountainous island of its size in the world. Thirty-five percent of its acreage is protected by world heritage and national park status. It boasts some of the best-preserved temperate forests left in the world. The coastline is stunning, with myriad coves, bays, beaches, estuaries, and spectacular cliffs. Tasmania is also a natural ark for many of Australia's unique mammals, birds, and alpine plants. (Those whose exposure to Tasmania has been limited to the Tasmanian Devil character from Warner Bros. Looney Tunes cartoons may be surprised to learn that such an animal really does exist; it's a carnivorous marsupial the size of a smallish dog.)

"I've ridden many tours in Tasmania," Richard Oddy began. "The scenery is spectacular and quite varied, the roads are very quiet (there are only 485,000 people on the whole island), and the automobile drivers you do encounter are very considerate to cyclists. Cycling is becoming more popular in Australia. Instead of being something people did because they couldn't afford a car, it's now something that people choose to do because they enjoy it. Since Tasmania is fairly small, someone who is relatively fit can circumnavigate the island in roughly two weeks, with a few rest days included. If you don't have that much time, I recommend riding from Launceston in the north, west through Cradle Mountain National Park, along the west coast to Strahan, and back across the island through Lake St. Clair National Park to the provincial capital of Hobart. No shuttles are necessary. You can ride out of Launceston on quiet roads and into downtown Hobart eight days later on a cycleway."

One of the highlights of any biking tour of Tasmania is a chance to come upon some of Australia's indigenous fauna. At your first stopover from Launceston, at Silver Ridge Retreat in Sheffield, you're likely to encounter the holy grail of Tassie critters—the platypus. These curious animals fuse facets from the reptile, bird, fish, and mammal families. They have fur, lay eggs, have a duckbill, a beaver-like tail, otter-like feet, use electro-perception to locate prey (like some fish); males are capable of delivering potent venom through a spur on their hind feet. While there's no consensus on the evolution of the platypus, Australian Aborigines believe the strange amalgamation resulted from a young female duck's disobedience: One day the duck strayed from her pond against the advice of her elders and swam down a stream. She climbed out on a patch of grass on the riverbank, unaware that this was the home of the lonely Water-rat. The Water-rat emerged, threatened her with his spear, and dragged her underground, where he forced her to mate. When the eggs hatched, the offspring had bills and four webbed feet, and fur instead of feathers, and on each hind leg they had a sharp spike like Water-rat's spear.

The route continues to Cradle Mountain-Lake St. Clair National Park. "This is a short day," Richard continued, "just 36 miles (58 km). We like to leave time whenever possible for riders to get off their bikes and take short hikes, and the area around majestic Cradle Mountain is certainly worth exploring. It's the beginning point of the Overland Track, one of the world's great hikes. One option is to hike around Dove Lake. Here, you have a very good chance of finding a few more of Australia's unique animals: wombats and wallabies." The flora in the park is also quite distinctive, particularly the pandani, which has a palmlike appearance. If you're feeling especially energetic, you can continue from Dove Lake up to the summit of craggy Cradle Mountain and look south out over much of the park. Next, you'll push through the isolated mountains of the west coast to the town of Strahan, above Macquarie Harbor. It's a long day—more than 90 miles (145 km) if you ride the entirety—but the mountain vistas are tremendous, and you feel exhilaration upon reaching the sea. Some will choose to rest a day in Strahan to stroll along the beach or take a boating excursion on the Gordon River—especially as the next day entails one of Tasmania's more invigorating and inspiring rides.

"The day from Strahan to Lake St. Clair—the southern end of Cradle Mountain–Lake St. Clair National Park—takes you through more superb mountain scenery," Richard described. "You head back inland through Queenstown. Several big climbs await. The first is leaving Queenstown en route to Lake Burbury. The next takes you over Victoria Pass, near the Franklin River, a favorite of white-water rafters. The last is King William Saddle, which takes you onto Tasmania's Central Plateau. I like to stop for a refreshment at one of the pubs in Derwent Bridge before pedaling the last few kilometers to our lodging at St. Clair Chalets. After nearly 88 miles (140 km), you've earned a pint." From here, the ride's intensity subsides. "There's a fantastic descent past more lakes and mountains into the town of Hamilton," Richard added. "I have such happy memories of the broad vistas of this stretch as I freewheel down gentle hills with no traffic to contend with."

RICHARD ODDY has had a passion for cycling for more than fifty years. This, combined with his love of travel, helped give birth to Pedaltours. When cyclists ask about a particular Pedaltours route, he can proudly say, "Yes, I have cycled that, climbed the hills, admired the views, and meandered through the valleys." Richard has biked in eighteen countries. He's commuted by bike for many years, has raced, and now tours by bike.

If You Go

► **Getting There:** The tour begins in Launceston and ends in Hobart. Both are served from Sydney and Melbourne by Qantas Air (800-227-4500; www.qantas.com).

► **Best Time to Visit:** The Aussie summer (January through April) sees lower rainfall and warmer temperatures in Tasmania.

► **Guides/Outfitters:** A number of outfitters lead trips around Tasmania, including Pedaltours (888-222-9187; www.pedaltours.co.nz).

► **Level of Difficulty:** This trip involves seven days of riding, with an average of 50 miles (80 km) a day. It's rated moderate to difficult.

► **Accommodations:** Richard recommends the following lodging options: in Sheffield, Silver Ridge Retreat (+61 3 6491 1727; www.sridge.com.au); in Cradle Mountain National Park, Cradle Mountain Lodge (+61 3 6492 2103; www.cradlemountainlodge.com.au); in Strahan, Strahan Village Cottages (+6471 7191; www.strahanvillage.com.au); in Lake St. Clair, St. Clair Chalets (+6289 1137); in Hamilton, Hamilton Hotel and B&Bs; in Hobart, Hotel Lenna (+61 3 6232 3900; www.lenna.com.au).

FLANDERS

RECOMMENDED BY **Joe Parkin**

"In 1985, I was living in northern California and had graduated from high school early so I could focus on bike racing," Joe Parkin began. "I got to know Bob Roll at that time. He was fresh off a trip to Europe, where he'd spent time racing in Switzerland and Italy. He and I hit it off, and he thought I had some potential as a racer. I was being courted by some semiprofessional teams, but was also thinking about college. Bob suggested that instead I go to Belgium. 'If you have skills, you'll know after six months over there,' he advised. 'If not, you'll figure out another plan.' I took his advice and worked three jobs to save money to make the trip. I left for Belgium in 1986, and by the second year I signed a contract with a pro team. Everything seemed larger than life—riding through fourteenth- or fifteenth-century towns like Bruges was astounding to a kid who'd grown up in subur-ban subdivisions. Also, bike racing was such a big part of the culture. Cycling was not very visible in the United States in the mid-'80s, but in Belgium bike racing *mattered*. In fact, in the spring and summer, you could find a professional race every day. It's called the *kermis* circuit; almost every town has a fair or *kermis*, and there's a race that goes along with it. Those first few years, I must have ridden 140 or 150 races each year!"

The Kingdom of Belgium is a small nation tucked between France, the Netherlands, Germany, and Luxembourg (an even smaller nation). Flanders, the northern section of the country, is primarily the domain of the Flemish people, Dutch-speaking Belgians. The southern region is known as Wallonia, and French is the primary language there. (Suffice it to say that there is no small amount of friction between the Flemish and Walloons.) Sitting astride the physical (and philosophical) border between the Germanic and Latin cultures, Belgium has frequently found its soil the site of armed conflicts staged by its larger neighbors (including World Wars I and II), earning it the unfortunate

31

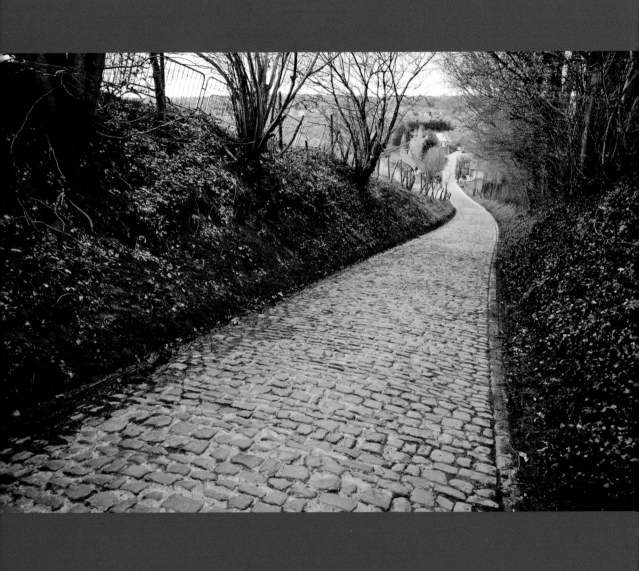

sobriquet "the battleground of Europe." Joe said, "It's been my experience that the people of Belgium are sometimes looked down upon by other western Europeans as being somehow 'backwoodsy,' or less sophisticated. I found them to be some of the friendliest people in Europe. In the cycling world, they take pride in being tough as nails, smiling through even the most grueling situations. Perhaps this comes from having to train in rain and sleet, perhaps from having endured so much warfare in their homeland. They seem to have developed a happy-go-lucky attitude that helps them get through."

Whether you're a hard-core racer or simply wish to ride in a beautiful setting, Flanders has something to offer. "For starters, the roads are beautiful, designed for cycling," Joe continued. "They are narrow, many with the famous Flemish cobblestones. The roads are quite interwoven. You might ride 20 miles (32 km) and not be more than 3 miles (4.8 km) from where you started.

"People are used to seeing bikes on the road, and you're not going to get honked at. Everyone bikes. On Sunday mornings, you'll see ladies all dolled up in heels and dresses, riding their bikes to the store to get groceries for Sunday dinner. If you have any mechanical troubles, chances are very good that a group of riders—or a motorist—will soon come by and help; and most everyone speaks English. From a ride-friendly perspective, the country is fairly flat. Not Holland flat, but flat enough that if you leave your fitness at home, you can still do a nice bike ride and not suffer. Many of the roads are tree-lined, so you can hide from the wind a bit. Flanders is very proud of its cycling history and heritage. There are plaques along the road denoting various climbs or pointing out that a road is part of the Tour of Flanders route. It's almost impossible to get lost, as there are directional signs everywhere. Wherever you stop, you'll find some wonderful baked goods and a good glass of beer. I recall that when I lived in Belgium, if you rode into a brewery on your bike, you were offered a free beer."

If you only have one chance to visit Flanders, you might consider a trip in the early spring, when Belgium becomes the epicenter of the bike-racing world. The Tour of Flanders has been running at the beginning of April since 1913, launched by a publisher named Karel Van Wijnendaele, who operated a sporting newspaper. Today, the one-day race covers approximately 155 miles (250 km); the course (and exact mileage) varies slightly year to year. "I remember watching the race on TV and seeing what seemed to be modest climbs," Joe recalled. "I thought, 'What's so hard about that?' When I competed, I understood. If you do a sustained climb in the Alps or Colorado, you're going to suffer

OPPOSITE:
The famed Koppenberg, a 22 percent grade, looks peaceful here. Add a few thousand riders and it's a different story.

for a while. Given the narrowness of the Tour of Flanders course (often no wider than two average sidewalks) and the number of cyclists, riding this event has the feeling of being in a bar fight that lasts seven hours. You have two hundred other cyclists going 35 miles per hour coming into a 90-degree turn that heads into a steep climb up a road the size of an alley, with everyone trying to be at one place at one time. I believe the Tour of Flanders is the hardest one-day race in the world, and I think there are many pros who would agree. [Perhaps the most illustrious climb is the Koppenberg, a 253-foot-high hill in the town of Oudenaarde. Part of the trail—notorious for its slippery cobblestones—has a 22 percent grade, and it's not uncommon for some riders to carry their bikes up the hill.] I can't overstate the importance of the race for Belgian cyclists. If you're a Belgian and you win, you will be remembered for this achievement for the rest of your life. You could go on to win the Tour de France or cure cancer, but in Belgium you'll always be known as the person who won the Tour of Flanders."

Joe recently had a chance to ride the Tour of Flanders again . . . and he almost turned it down! "I was visiting Flanders on a press trip," he continued, "and there's an open cyclist sportif the day before when anyone can ride the course. You have the option of doing 62 miles (100 km), 100 miles (160 km), or the entire course. Anyone who considers themselves a cyclist and finds themselves anywhere near Belgium the first weekend in April just has to go and do this ride. The media group I was traveling with planned to do the middle portion of the ride. I remembered it from riding the race twenty years before, and when they asked if I wanted to go, I said, 'Hell no! That's the hardest ride I've ever done, and I don't need to suffer through that again.' Eventually I gave in, and it was a truly incredible experience. There are something like nineteen thousand people who pay money to ride this course during the sportif. You'll have some people there on $15,000 carbon fiber bikes; you'll also have seventy-year-old men riding bikes they used to race in the 1960s. Even more amazing, you have people lining the racecourse cheering on the sportif riders. It's one thing to have people attending a professional race, but to have crowds out cheering on Joe Public is amazing. These riders aren't out for money or glory; they're just out for personal accomplishment. The Belgians appreciate that you're out there pushing for something more substantial than planting yourself on the couch and channel surfing."

JOE PARKIN was an amateur bike racer in California when he met Bob Roll, who advised him to move to Belgium to further his cycling career. He represented the United States at the World Professional Cycling Championships and the Cyclo-cross World Championships. Following his road-racing years in Belgium, he returned to the United States and began a successful second career as a pro mountain bike racer. Joe then launched a third career as a bicycling journalist. His book *A Dog in a Hat: An American Bike Racer's Story of Mud, Drugs, Blood, Betrayal, and Beauty in Belgium* chronicles his time on the Belgium circuit; his second book, *Come and Gone: A True Story of Blue-Collar Bike Racing in America,* looks at his time as a mountain bike racer. Today, Joe serves as editor of *Bike* and *Paved* magazines.

If You Go

▶ **Getting There:** You'll want to fly to Brussels, which is served by many international carriers. Joe recommends limiting your time here!

▶ **Best Time to Visit:** If you're a racer, you'll want to visit during the first week of April, when the Tour of Flanders is held. Mid-April to mid-October is considered to be in season.

▶ **Guides/Outfitters:** A number of tour operators lead trips to attend the Tour of Flanders, including Velo Classic Tours (212-779-9599; www.veloclassic.com) and Bike Belgium (720-295-0758; www.bikebelgium.com).

▶ **Level of Difficulty:** Moderate . . . unless you ride the Tour of Flanders course, which is difficult. Tours generally entail five to six days of riding.

▶ **Accommodations:** Oudenaarde is one of the centers of Flanders's bicycling activity, and the city's website (www.oudenaarde.be) lists lodging options.

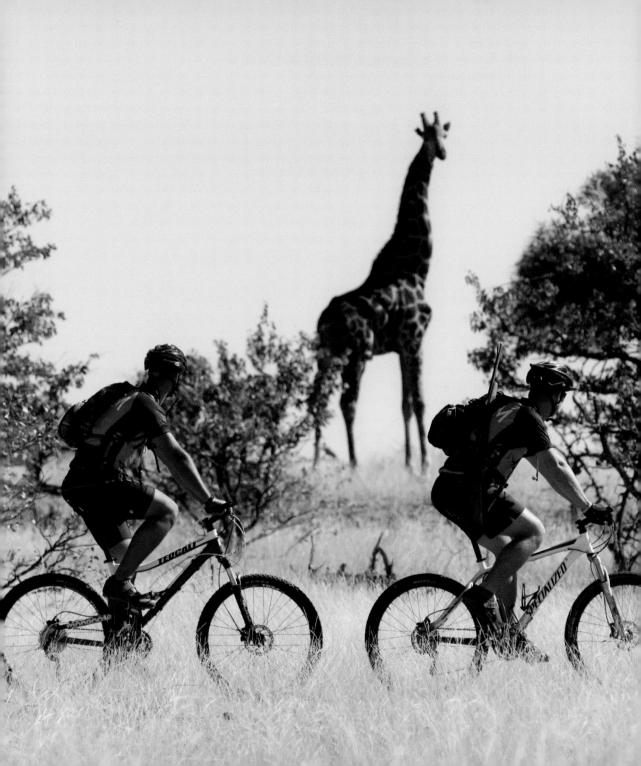

TOUR DE TULI

RECOMMENDED BY **Joe Kurmaskie**

Traveling cyclists are used to encountering road surfaces of varying types and quality. It might be a well-paved bike lane in Portland or Manhattan, a wooden train trestle in British Columbia or South Dakota, or a gravel trail in Switzerland. In the Mapungubwe region of southern Africa, it's likely to be ancient elephant trails . . . with modern-day elephants alive and well and sometimes foraging along the route.

Welcome to the Tour de Tuli!

"From the moment I'd heard about the tour, it had become one of those irresistible but ultimately inexplicable impulses cyclists are prone to," Joe "Metal Cowboy" Kurmaskie explained. "A bit into the trip—as I watched a herd of zebra approach a clean-running water hole that my group of cyclists was cooling off in—I realized why I'd come. It was to own a few of my life's moments again. The trip had called to me because it allowed me to stay out on trails from first light until the shine of a fat moon guided me, dirty, spent, overwhelmed, and blissful, into camp. It also took place in a daunting, remarkable landscape that was burning itself into my seen-it-all brain."

The Tour de Tuli is a one-of-a-kind bike adventure that takes riders through the greater Mapungubwe region, an area of open savanna around the confluence of the Limpopo and Shashe Rivers that encompasses parts of eastern Botswana, southern Zimbabwe, and northeastern South Africa. (Fort Tuli, incidentally, is the midpoint of the ride and the site of one of the early British colonial outposts in Zimbabwe, circa 1890.) Over the course of four or five days (depending on the year), it takes you 45 to 50 miles (70 to 80 km) each day along rough trails (literal elephant paths) through lush riparian woodlands, across rivers, up water-carved creases of sandstone hills, and through border checkpoints (Joe remembered one enforced by a matronly woman at a card table jammed into the

OPPOSITE:
Giraffes are the
tallest onlookers
you'll encounter
on the wild and
wooly Tour
de Tuli.

loose sand on the banks of the Limpopo River, she was only armed with an ink pad and a basket of pomegranates; no fruit was offered as Joe's passport was stamped). The introductory packet says it all: "Please register only if you have a SENSE OF ADVENTURE and are happy to accept the unexpected!" The tour—which draws upward of four hundred visitors most years, divided into groups of roughly twenty riders—was conceived to raise funds for Children in the Wilderness, a nonprofit environmental and life skills educational program that exposes the youth of southern Africa to their wildlife heritage and to the virtues of sustained community and conservation partnerships.

The Kingdom of Mapungubwe was one of southern Africa's most developed civilizations in the thirteenth century, with a thriving gold and ivory trade with Egypt, India, and China; it was a predecessor to the Kingdom of Zimbabwe. Archaeological sites, including Mapungubwe Hill and K2, reflect the region's rich cultural past. The area also includes several national parks—Mapungubwe National Park and Northern Tuli Game Reserve, which are home to much of the fauna safari visitors seek to encounter, including elephant, giraffe, white rhino, eland, gemsbok, as well as more elusive predators like lions, leopards, and hyenas. On Joe's first day of riding, local residents were certainly making their presence known. "The elephants seemed more bemused than riled up by our presence on their trails," he recounted. "The giraffes simply turned their necks in slow motion to take a second look. The warthogs scattered like quail flushed from hiding. Every time three or four darted among the bikes in our pack, our guide reminded us that if one rider went down, the rest had to push on—bush rules. Logical. Maybe necessary. But a little harsher than one might have expected of a charity ride."

If marauding warthogs don't provide enough drama, perhaps the presence of gun-toting guides and soldiers will up the ante. "In photos I'd seen of previous tours, bandanna-masked guides wearing carbines slung across their shoulders like messenger bags emerged Mad Max–style through the kicked-up dust of elephant trails," Joe described. "I asked one of our guides, Sarah, where her gun was. 'I think a guide shot himself in the foot a few years ago,' she said, 'so now we use elephant bangers, a can that sounds like a gunshot when you pop it. Besides, the animals have thousands of miles of open country to get away. Guns are false security. And they would only piss off President Mugabe.' As we rode through the most remote stretches of the bush—'the back of beyond,' it's called—we repeatedly came upon skin-and-bone soldiers propped against shepherd trees, posted by Mugabe and the Zimbabwean government to monitor our passage. Out of empathy, not pity or threat, we gave them food. They had us hold their rusty weapons so they could balance plates on their pointy knees while we coached them not to eat too fast."

Seeing elephants in the wild is one of the thrills that any visitor to Africa hopes to experience. One day, Joe got a little more pachyderm excitement than he'd bargained for. "We passed a herd of sixty or seventy elephants. By the time we got there, they'd had put up with hundreds of cyclists pedaling by their feeding grounds. Suddenly, the warthogs weren't the most dangerous beasts on the trail. As our group rolled by, a twelve-thousand-pounder began waving its ears repeatedly and throwing sand in all directions. I was one of the final riders trying to slip past when it charged. Elephants can go from 0 to 25 mph in short order. Someone caught the elephant's first burst of speed on video—and its deafening roar and the pause as it seemed to sink down on itself, stockpiling kinetic dynamite for what I felt certain would be a closing stamp of death. The video failed to capture my schoolgirl scream of terror. The oft-cited phenomenon of everything slowing down during a life-threatening situation didn't play out for me. I was in a blur of thoughtless primal fear until I was well beyond the herd. Then I was conscious only of breathing, though in ragged gasps.

"Later the locals would tell me that the elephant's behavior was a mock charge, that if the animal had really meant business, it would have tucked in its trunk so as not to damage its vital equipment, and would have led with its tusks. With not a little amusement, they reminded me that the hyenas that had trapped me inside a Porta Potty the previous evening (where I'd managed a fitful, seated sleep against the bathroom's wall) had actually been a more formidable threat."

JOE KURMASKIE, dubbed the "Metal Cowboy" by a blind rancher he encountered one icy morning in Idaho, has been addicted to the intoxicating freedom and power of the bicycle ever since he "borrowed" his big sister's banana-seat bike at the age of five. As he careened down the neighborhood hill, much to his parents' dismay, Joe set in motion what has become a lifelong love affair with the road and the wheel. Joe has been a journalist for two decades. He's been a contributing writer to *Bicycling*, *Details*, and *Men's Journal*. He worked as an editor for five years at an AP newspaper before becoming an author and entertainer (mostly so he could sleep in later). His work has also appeared in *Details*, *Bike Midwest*, and the *San Francisco Chronicle*. He reviews books for *The Oregonian* and is an educator for Literary Arts Inc and Community of Writers (COW) writer in residence at Portland State University. Joe's books include *Metal Cowboy, Riding Between the Lines,* and *Momentum Is Your Friend.* He lives in Portland, Oregon, with his wife and four boys.

If You Go

► **Getting There:** The trip begins and ends around Mapungubwe National Park. Johannesburg, roughly 300 miles away, has the closest international airport and is served by many carriers.

► **Best Time to Visit:** The Tour de Tuli is generally held the first week in August.

► **Guides/Outfitter:** The ride is orchestrated by Tour de Wilderness (+27 0 11 8071800; www.tourdewilderness.com) to raise funds for Children in the Wilderness (www .childreninthewilderness.com).

► **Level of Difficulty:** Extreme—and even tougher if you encounter charging elephants. The event unfolds over six days, and entails 35 miles (60 km) to 50 miles (80 km) each day.

► **Accommodations:** During the tour, you'll sleep in comfortable tents. Options for Johannesburg are highlighted on the city's website (www.joburg.org.za).

OKANAGAN VALLEY

RECOMMENDED BY **David Baker**

British Columbia's Okanagan Valley—midway between the Canadian Rockies to the east and the Pacific to the west—has been called the "Napa of the North." Nestled in a rain shadow between the Coastal and Monashee ranges, the Okanagan sees very little precipitation—especially for British Columbia. Little rain combined with warm summer temperatures and many microclimates have fostered a thriving wine industry, with more than 160 wineries operating in the region as of this writing. However, for David Baker, the Okanagan's appeal as a bicycling destination goes beyond its wines. "The weather that makes for great wine growing is certainly attractive, but the Okanagan also has a strong cycling culture," he began. "The valley is the site of Ironman Canada, one of the longest-running Ironman competitions in North America. The race here is a qualifier for the world championship, and it brings many top athletes out on the roads. Some of the rides in the Okanagan take you on the rails of the Kettle Valley Railroad, which played a significant role in the settling of the Canadian West. In the Okanagan you get forest, vineyards, and desert in a shifting palette of textures, often framed by sweeping mountain or lake vistas."

The Okanagan Valley runs approximately 100 miles (160 km), from the town of Kelowna in the north to the village of Osoyoos in the south (just above the U.S. border); Okanagan Lake runs much of the length of the valley. David likes to move north to south, mixing wine tasting with "rail-to-trail" rides and opportunities to cool off in one of the region's many lakes. Using Manteo Resort as a base, a perfect first ride will take you into the hills above Kelowna. You might stop for lunch at Summerhill Pyramid Winery's Sunset Organic Bistro, which serves up fabulous views of Okanagan Lake and the surrounding mountains as well as wild and organic fare (featuring produce grown on-site)

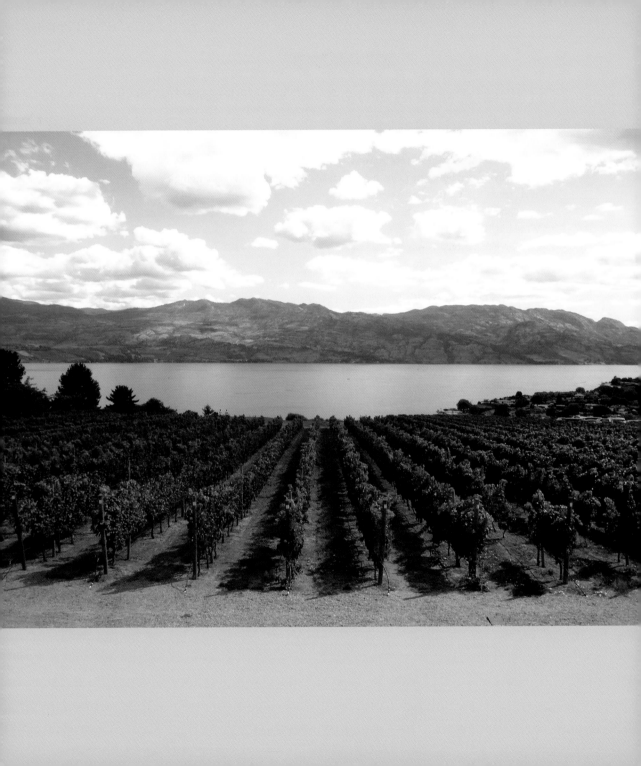

and Summerhill's award-winning, organic wines, including Cipes Brut, a sparkling wine fashioned from Riesling and Chardonnay grapes. "The winery has a large pyramid (painstakingly designed and built by owner Stephen Cipes) that's used to house the wines—particularly the sparkling wines," David continued. "It's central to the proprietor's vision for the winery." After a few more miles, you'll visit Carmelis Goat Cheese Artisan Inc., a family-owned boutique goat cheese maker that creates varieties ranging from traditional chèvre to a Camembert-style cheese to "Goatgonzola"—a blue cheese, of course!

The Okanagan wine industry, it's worth noting, has had a bumpy ride to respectability. Wine has been made in the valley since European settlers arrived in the early 1800s, though the early product—pressed from native grape species—had, well, an acquired taste. Early efforts to cultivate European (Vinifera) grape varieties failed, but changes in governance concerning wine production and perseverance paid off. The microclimates David mentioned allow significantly different varietals to be grown in close proximity to each other. New cultivation techniques have yielded not only high-quality Rieslings, Gewürztraminers, and Pinot Gris (the Okanagan rests at the same latitude as Germany's Mosel Valley), but Pinot Noirs, Cabernet Sauvignons, and Merlots as well.

David mentioned several wineries he enjoys sharing with guests. "For pure spectacle, it's hard to beat Mission Hill. From the grandeur of the buildings to the majestic views looking out over the valley, it's over the top. For a unique wine, you can't miss Silver Sage. They do a variety of fruit wines, but their most memorable wine is a Gewürztraminer flavored with sage. You can't help but think that this is the wine that *must* be served with turkey at Thanksgiving. I also enjoy Church and State Wines, particularly their tasting area. You sit at a long bar. Behind the bar, there's a wall of glass with wine barrels on display behind. The glass reflects the vineyards behind you. It's a wonderful montage. Overall, the tasting experience in the Okanagan is very relaxed. Vintners are easygoing and have a sense of humor, but are still eager to educate visitors about what they're doing."

A "must-ride" for any cyclist touring the Okanagan region is a portion of the Kettle Valley Railtrail. The railway has an interesting provenance. Up until the later 1800s, western Canada was quite isolated from the eastern portion of the country. It was well-known that there were rich mineral reserves in present-day south central British Columbia. Canada's first transcontinental railroad, the Canadian Pacific Railway, was significantly north of the mining reserves and of little use in getting mining supplies in

OPPOSITE:
Some think
of British
Columbia's
Okanagan Valley
as the "Napa
of the North."

or minerals out. Many Americans were coming across the border to mine silver, with the Northern Pacific Railroad and its station in Spokane acting as the commercial hub. Canadian authorities recognized that they were losing a great deal of revenue, and plans to build a new rail line to connect the interior with Vancouver—which would become the Kettle Valley Railroad—were put in motion. The line was especially notable for its trestles that bridged several of the region's gaping canyons. Completed in 1915 (and considered one of the more costly lines per mile built in North America), the line carried freight until the early 1960s and passengers until the early 1970s, when it was closed to train traffic. "The railway bed never has a slope of more than 2.2 percent and was away from roads, and people realized that it was great for hiking and biking," David explained. "But it was in disrepair—especially the trestles. The Canadian government stepped in and made improvements in 2003, but that summer, terrific forest fires damaged many of the trestles. The government stepped in again and rebuilt the trestles to have the same look and feel.

"One of my favorite sections of the Kettle Valley Railtrail (which stretches more than 350 miles [560 km]) is Myra Canyon. There are eighteen trestles—and several tunnels—to traverse the canyon. One of the trestles (over Bellevue Creek) is more than 656 feet long and 213 feet high. Riding over that canyon, you get a feel for all the engineering that went into getting the railways established in the region. Another wonderful section of the trail goes along Skaha Lake and ends near Okanagan Falls. You're along the water all day. There's a nice beach near the end where you can wade in and cool off."

DAVID BAKER owned and operated an engineering firm that designed wind turbine facilities throughout North America. He sold his company in 2008 and left the corporate world the following year. He had cycled throughout his youth (even through the snowy Calgary winters) and kept his 1978 Sekine 10 speed for thirty years. After a couple of tours as a client with DuVine Adventures, it was clear to him that guiding would be a perfect fit for his next challenge—organizing, riding, and sharing Canada as a DuVine guide! David lives with his wife, Barb, in the Okanagan Valley in the summer and Mexico in the winter.

If You Go

▶ **Getting There:** Most visitors fly into Kelowna, which is served from Vancouver and Toronto by Air Canada (888-247-2262; www.aircanada.com) and WestJet (888-937-8538; www.westjet.com).

▶ **Best Time to Visit:** The weather is most bike-friendly from mid-May through September. September is David's favorite month to ride—"Less crowded and the end of the month is the beginning of the crush!"

▶ **Guides/Outfitters:** DuVine Adventures Bicycle Tours (888-396-5383; www.duvine .com) leads tours around the Okanagan.

▶ **Level of Difficulty:** The itinerary above involves four days of riding, ranging from 18 to 32 miles (29 to 51 km) per day. It's rated moderate.

▶ **Accommodations:** In Kelowna, David recommends Manteo Resort (800-445-5255; www.manteo.com); in Osoyoos, Walnut Beach Resort (877-936-5400; www.walnutbeach osoyoos.com).

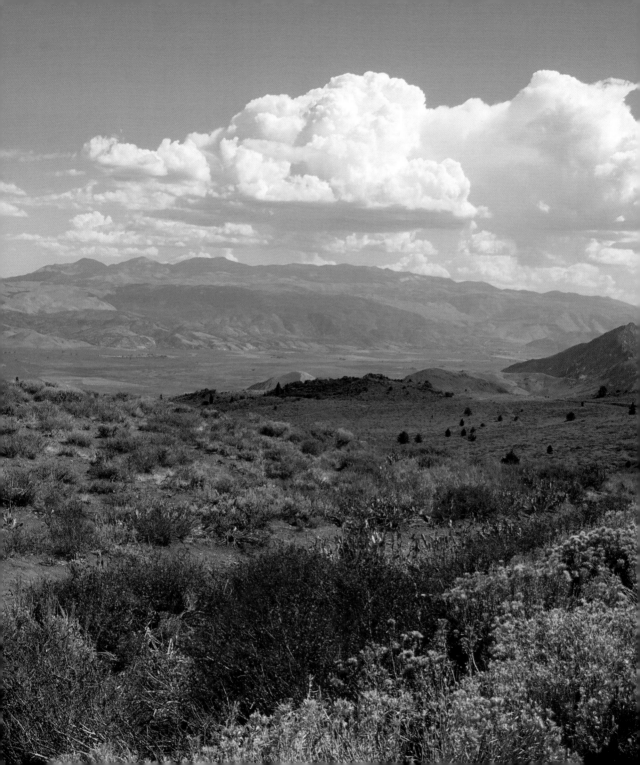

EASTERN SIERRAS

RECOMMENDED BY **Arlen Hall**

"I have always been intrigued by the Sierras, at least in part because I've always wanted to visit Yosemite," Arlen Hall began. "I biked across the range from west to east as part of a cross-country ride I completed a few years back, but I'd never ridden it north to south. I recently had a chance to do so. I have to admit that I didn't think it would be as magnificent as it was. I've ridden more than 40,000 miles, and I don't think any of the rides I've done were as consistently stunning as this one. There is some serious climbing in the eastern Sierras, enough to be a challenge for most intermediate riders. But when you get to the top, you're treated to vistas that are truly majestic. Even in August or September, you're looking out at snowcapped mountains framed against cobalt-blue skies. After those climbs you're treated to a sensational descent."

"The range of light"—that's what naturalist John Muir called the Sierra Nevadas, a vast granite range that rises east of California's central valley and extends to Nevada, stretching some 400 miles north to south. Arlen's ride focuses on the northern portion of the Sierras' eastern escarpment, beginning in Truckee and moving south toward Mammoth Lakes. You'll have a day around Truckee to get acclimated to the altitude (nearly 6,000 feet; some passes on the trip will take you above 9,000). A favorite warm-up ride takes you around scenic Donner Lake, named for the ill-fated party of settlers who stayed near it in the winter of 1846–47, some of whom resorted to cannibalism to avoid starvation. But don't worry: No matter how challenging a warm-up you undertake, starvation should not be an issue. Truckee, a bustling four-season resort town, has many fine eating options. If you're traveling with Adventure Cycling, a catered meal will await you in your campground. "A caterer travels with the group with a portable kitchen," Arlen explained. "Each dinner on the trip is exquisite."

OPPOSITE:
The ride from
Truckee to the
Mammoth Lakes
region along the
eastern spine
of the Sierra
Nevada offers
up consistently
stunning views.

From Truckee, you'll head along the Truckee River toward Lake Tahoe, passing Squaw Valley (home of the 1960 Winter Olympics) and Tahoe City en route. (At Tahoe City, you might pause at Fanny Bridge to peer down at the immense rainbow trout that gather here at the lake's outlet to feed on snacks proffered by visitors. If you're thirsty, grab a beer at The Bridgetender, where you can watch the tourists watching the trout!) Much of your afternoon will be spent pedaling along the western shore of North America's largest alpine lake (and second deepest, at 1,645 feet)—amazingly blue and clear. "Near the end of the day toward the southern end of the lake, there's a spot called Inspiration Point," Arlen continued. "You're 1,000 feet above Emerald Bay, which has Lake Tahoe's only island, Fannette Island. It's sublime." The next day takes you farther south, through the aspen and pine forests of Hope Valley, past the town of Markleeville, and on to Topaz Lake in Nevada. "This is no doubt the hardest day on the trip," Arlen said. "We have two significant passes to traverse, first Luther Pass (at 7,700 feet) and then Monitor Pass (at 8,300 feet). The climb to Monitor is 12 miles (19 km), with grades that range from 6 to 12 percent. A few of our riders needed the support van that day, but once you reach the summit, there's a 10-mile (16 km) descent to the lake, where we camp that evening."

Day four takes you farther along the escarpment to the small resort town of Lee Vining, on the shores of Mono Lake. As you roll through Bridgeport Valley, the peaks that form the boundary of Yosemite come into view . . . but better rewards await, as you make the climb up Conway Summit to partake of the view over Mono Lake and beyond. "You're 1,500 feet above the lake," Arlen described. "You can see the little town of Lee Vining to the west, and you can make out the mineral growths that protrude from the lake. From here, it's an 11-mile (17 km) scream down to the town, with the lake and the Minaret Range in view." Mono Lake is a saline body of water that provides a sanctuary for millions of migratory shorebirds. It gained notoriety in the 1970s as scientists realized that water diversions from the upper sections of the Mono basin (engineered by the Los Angeles Department of Water & Power) were bringing the lake to dangerously low levels. A court battle ensued, with Mono Lake supporters prevailing; water levels have been consistently rising since 1994. After the previous day's 79 miles (127 km), day five provides an opportunity to relax. Some may choose to "rest" by cycling up to Tioga Pass, which sits at 9,900 feet—a 3,000-plus-foot climb. From here, you can continue into the eastern section of Yosemite National Park. You also have the option of driving into Yosemite, or to the nearby ghost town of Bodie, a former gold mining boomtown . . . or merely reclining by the lake.

After the layover at Mono Lake, you'll climb back into the Sierras and make your way to the resort area of Mammoth Lakes. En route, you'll ride the June Lake Loop, pause at Oh! Ridge (the exclamation speaks to the splendor of the mountains behind June Lake), and climb to Deadman's Summit (8,400 feet), before descending to Mammoth. This is a shorter day in the saddle, in part to leave time to enjoy the many other recreational amenities the region has to offer—mountain biking, fishing, boating, or a soak in Mammoth Hot Creek. "Another thing I love about the eastern Sierras is the abundance of non-biking activities at just about every stop," Arlen said. "There are so many lakes along the way, there's always a chance to take a swim." You'll have another layover day at Mammoth, though many will opt to ride. One route takes you to the Minaret Summit, which looks out over the Ansel Adams Wilderness and the eastern edge of Yosemite. From here, you can continue on to Devils Postpile National Monument, a remarkable display of columnar basalt. "There's another ride I like to do," Arlen continued. "It takes you up a steep pass to the Rock Creek Lakes Resort and Pie in the Sky Café. The climb to the pass is 8 miles (12 km), and the grade goes from 8 to 10 percent, but at the top, a host of homemade pies are waiting—boysenberry, cheddar pear, rhubarb, and pecan chocolate chip among them. I'm on a quest to find the best coconut cream pie on earth, so that's what I chose.

"I have to admit that I'm not much of a hammerhead," Arlen added. "I'm a big guy, and climbing mountain passes is not my favorite bicycling activity. I can and will do it, though it's not my first choice. When I was riding through the eastern Sierras, I forgot about the effort it took to make those climbs, because I would look up and see those majestic vistas. The mountains would give me pause and make me consider what a little creature I am in the context of this big world. The view at Inspiration Point did this, as did the view at Conway Summit, my visit to Yosemite, and the ride up to Pie in the Sky."

ARLEN HALL is Adventure Cycling's tours director. He joined the Adventure Cycling team in August 2011, relocating from Putnam, Connecticut. In addition to leading tours for Adventure Cycling since 2005, he has logged more than 40,000 miles leading trips for middle school and high school teens since 1998. He has also served as tours director of two nonprofit organizations, 10thGear and BIKETERNITY, while running his own computer software company, Rainbow Software Solutions. Arlen has cycled coast to coast on four occasions, three times with teens. In 2007, he was touched by the stories of boys afflicted with Duchenne muscular dystrophy and has led charity rides, called JettRides, for the Jett Foundation of Kingston, Massachusetts, ever since. Arlen loves pie and is currently searching, by bicycle, for the Best Coconut Cream Pie in America. He rides, eats, and enjoys watching his two adult sons, Chris and Brandon, find their own way in life.

If You Go

▶ **Getting There:** This ride begins and ends in Truckee, California, which is easily reached from the Reno-Tahoe International Airport served by most major carriers.

▶ **Best Time to Visit:** Roads in the eastern Sierras should be clear from mid-June to mid-October.

▶ **Guides/Outfitters:** The ride described here is led by Adventure Cycling Association (800-755-2453; www.adventurecycling.org).

▶ **Level of Difficulty:** This itinerary entails six days of riding, averaging 45 miles (72 km) per day. It's rated moderate to difficult.

▶ **Accommodations:** Adventure Cycling trips are generally camping-oriented. You'll find a list of lodging options in towns along the route at Visit California (www.visitcalifornia .com).

WINE COUNTRY

RECOMMENDED BY **Jonathan Hershberger**

"I tend to think in pictures, and when I think of the Wine Country, the first picture that comes to mind is the sunrise," Jonathan Hershberger led off. "It's a procession of cool pastels as you wake up and the clouds and mist begin to fade away with the rising sun. That image is augmented by the 'whoosh' of hot air balloons rising and the rustle of other riders waking up to start their day. The mornings are cool and crisp—a great way to start your day on the bike. As the day proceeds, the temperatures warm, and the smells are enticing and robust—especially in the fall during the grape crush. The roads are gradual and forgiving in the valleys for the novice cyclist; hard-core riders can find great climbs in the mountains that define each valley. The food here is phenomenal. And of course, there's the wine."

California's Sonoma and Napa Valleys—an hour or so north and east of San Francisco—seem to have been created solely for the delight of the pedaling gastronome. Boutique wineries, award-winning restaurants, and sumptuous inns are situated at intervals that accommodate a wide range of riders, all set against landscapes of rolling vineyards, gentle mountains, and even a majestic redwood forest. A mild Mediterranean-style climate tops it all off. With seven-hundred-plus wineries between Sonoma and Napa—and as of this writing, fourteen Michelin-starred eateries—a plethora of itineraries awaits.

"There are three wineries that I especially like to visit on a tour. The first is Cakebread Cellars (in the town of Rutherford, in Napa). Most people know of this winery, which produces a number of fine wines, including Cabernet Sauvignons, Chardonnays, and Sauvignon Blancs. The next is Summit Lake Vineyards, which is at elevation (about 2,000 feet above the valley floor) on Howell Mountain. (The cooler microclimate here produces fine Cabs and Zinfandels.) Summit is a smaller operation run by the Brakeman

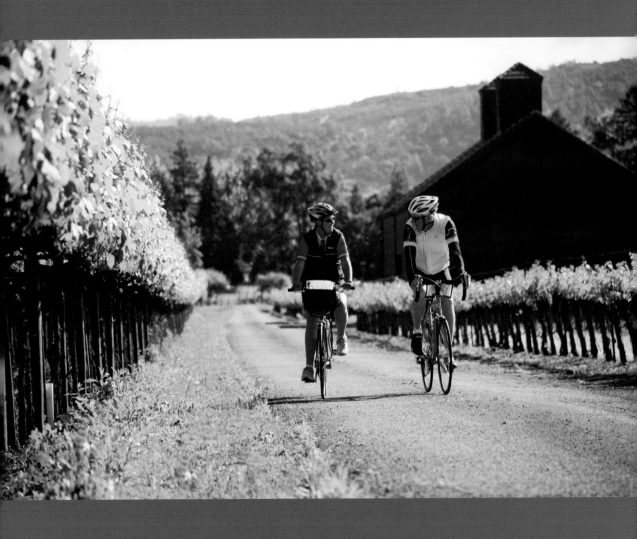

family—Bob and his daughter Heather. They have horses and chickens on the property and a golden retriever named Cody that loves to play fetch. It's a bit of a climb to get up there, but once people arrive, they don't want to leave. It's a place of peace. My other favorite is Arista Winery in Sonoma on the Russian River, which is known for its Pinot Noirs. This is another family operation, and members of the McWilliams clan are usually on hand to do tours and tastings.

"The personal touch makes these and other Wine Country venues special. It's one thing to taste a wine at the bar. It's another to be taken back into the picnic area and get a personalized tasting with the owners. By getting a chance to meet the winemakers, you have the opportunity to be educated about the vintages. This way you have something to bring back home and share beyond a glass of Cabernet. Many of the region's wineries have picnic areas, and there are many places—from Oakville Grocery Store to Jimtown General Store—where you can pick up sandwiches, lettuce wraps, and olives to enjoy with a glass of wine in those sanctums. These are the perfect places to relax—no humidity, no bugs. You can eat, energize, and get back on your bike to ride."

As night falls and the air begins to soften and cool, thoughts drift to the dinner table. You could do worse than Thomas Keller's celebrated eateries—the French Laundry and Bouchon. A few others that Jonathan likes to visit are Hurley's (in Yountville) and Madrona Manor (in Healdsburg). "Hurley's sometimes serves a wild braised boar with hearty vegetables and a soft polenta—a great comfort food. They also serve an exquisite ice cream sandwich with hints of raspberry and chocolate. Madrona Manor serves a three- or five-course wine-paired meal. Each course is prepared to fuse with the wine. By the time guests are done with the meal, they've had an education in wine and food pairing. It's like adding one to one and getting three."

With all of Wine Country's convivial trappings, it's easy to forget that there's some great cycling to be had here as well. "Two rides jump to mind for scenery," Jonathan continued. "One is the route that leads from Sonoma into Napa. You cycle through the Carneros region, and then head up the Oakville Grade. Forested land gives way to more arid, brown country. As you start your descent into Napa by St. Helena, the whole valley stretches out before you, this verdant land of abundance. It almost radiates. Over in Sonoma, a favorite ride takes you through the Russian River valley, past the town of Guerneville, and into the Armstrong Redwoods. It's amazing to see these giant trees— the tallest is more than 300 feet, and the oldest dates back to AD 600. Your whole world

OPPOSITE:
With over
seven hundred
wineries and
fourteen Michelin-
starred eateries,
California's
Wine Country
was created for
the pedaling
gastronome.

quiets down here. You can almost hear the trees speak. If you want to get your heart rate going, Wine Country has climbs too. Trinity Road (in Napa) has an 18 to 20 percent grade, and Sweetwater Springs boasts a 20 percent grade. They will kick most people's butts!

"Looking through the picture album in my head, I come back to a challenging morning ride, when I was biking with some friends," Jonathan mused. "You're working hard, you're tired, you're sweating, but your friends are rooting you on, and you're rooting for anyone who's behind you. Finally, you arrive at the winery that's your lunch spot. You share sandwiches, salad, and the vintner brings you a glass of wine. The sky is brilliantly blue overhead and you're breaking bread with friends, a real celebration of life."

JONATHAN HERSHBERGER has been leading and guiding trips in the California Wine Country since 2001. In 2005, he joined the staff of Trek Travel and became their trip expert in the region. His passions for traveling, good food, fine wine, stellar chocolate, and exercise have taken him all over the globe. Currently Jonathan splits the year between Vail Resorts in Colorado, where he is a guide and instructor during the winter months, and Trek Travel, where he leads trips during the summer months. You can find Jonathan leading trips for Trek Travel anywhere between northern California and western Europe.

If You Go

▶ **Getting There:** Guests generally fly into San Francisco and shuttle to Napa/Sonoma.

▶ **Best Time to Visit:** Dry, sunny weather is fairly reliable from May through October; days are a bit warmer in the summer months, though it always cools down at night.

▶ **Guides/Outfitters:** Companies leading trips through Wine Country include Trek Travel (866-464-8735; www.trektravel.com) and Backroads (800-462-2848; www.backroads.com).

▶ **Level of Difficulty:** This itinerary entails six days of riding, roughly 30 miles (48 km) a day. It's rated moderate.

▶ **Accommodations:** There are fine inns and resorts all over Wine Country. A few Jonathan recommends are MacArthur Place in Sonoma (707-938-2929; www.macarthurplace.com), Vintage Inn in Yountville (707-944-1112; www.vintageinn.com), and Madrona Manor (707-433-4231; www.madronamanor.com).

ARENAL TO GUANACASTE

RECOMMENDED BY **Ronald Calvo**

Costa Rica is much celebrated for its natural beauty, access to both the Caribbean and the Pacific, its abundance of habitat—from tropical rain forest and mountains to cloud forest—and even more for its farsightedness. "Why would we cut down a tree and sell it once when we could keep it standing and sell it over and over again?" Costa Rican President Rodrigo Carazo Odio said in the late 1970s. This ethos has led to the preservation of large swaths of the country's interior (some 23 percent) and a progressive attitude toward the possibilities of ecotourism.

"There are so many different landscapes, changes in topography (from sea level to 13,000 feet) and microclimates," Ronald Calvo began. "With just 0.03 percent of the planet's territory (Costa Rica is the size of West Virginia), it has 7 percent of the world's biodiversity. You may see two or three very different Costa Ricas in a single day's ride, and every trip is different. When I originally set out to create this trip, I envisioned six full days of biking. But given that our tropical climate might make that schedule a bit tough for some people—and given the many other incredible outdoor adventure opportunities Costa Rica has to offer—we combined some into an excursion that moves west from the Caribbean slope, across the continental divide at Lake Arenal, then on to Guanacaste (Gold Coast) on the northern Pacific coast."

What gets your heart pumping: White-water rapids? Active volcanoes? Immaculate beaches? A ride across Costa Rica won't disappoint. A half-day float trip on the Pacuare River—considered one of the world's great white-water rivers—is a splendid introduction to the rain forest. Over the span of 14 miles (22 km), you'll pass through untrammeled rain forest habitat that can only be reached by raft. This stretch covers the Pacuare's biggest rapids—Dos Montanas, Cimarron, Upper and Lower Huacas—and passes thirteen

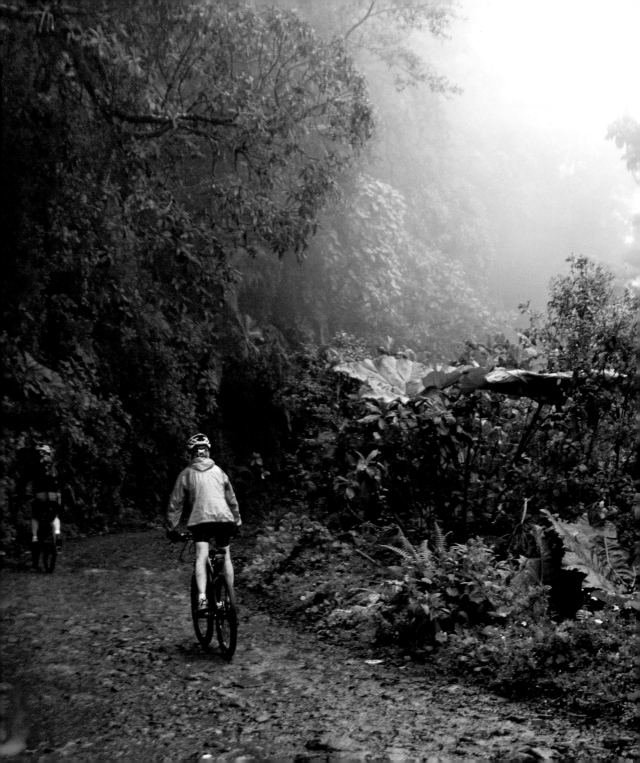

waterfalls. "Wildlife abounds in the surrounding rain forest," Ronald said, "though some creatures, including jaguar and black panther, are very seldom seen. We do sometimes see three-toed sloths hanging from the trees, and toucans. There's a group of indigenous people—the Cabecar—that live on a reservation nearby, and sometimes we see them down on the river. The water is cool but not unbearably so, and a swim can be quite refreshing—or even a surf through some of the milder rapids."

From the river, it's off to Arenal Volcano National Park, where you'll have a very good chance to see the workings of a live volcano—from a safe vantage point! Arenal is Costa Rica's most active volcano and has been consistently emitting lava since 1968. "Only three people out of every ten million around the world have seen flowing lava," Ronald continued, "and at Arenal, you can be one of those folks. There have been times when I've been riding in the region and have heard the rumbling of the volcano, or have come around a curve to see a mushroom cloud rising from the crater. There's a spot where we can drive where you're almost sure to see lava flowing down the slope of Arenal. It's a fabulous expression of Mother Nature's power." While here, you'll want to ride around Lake Arenal. "There's a nice combination of rolling hills and flats as you circle the lake," Ronald described. "The area has pineapple, banana, and heart-of-palm plantations—heart of palm, served with tortillas, refried beans, cheese, and a mild pico de gallo is one of our favorite lunches.

"On the latter part of that ride, the path is adjacent to the rain forest. Sometimes you're riding along and can hear the music of toucans and howler monkeys. The call of the howler monkeys is very loud and unsettling—I've had guests mistake it for that of a gorilla! But don't worry, there are no gorillas in Costa Rica . . . or the Western Hemisphere! We may round a corner to a clearing in the forest and come upon a troop of howlers, or have a toucan fly in front of us. There are 878 species of birds in Costa Rica—10 percent of the world's total species. I always bring a spyglass along in case I hear the call of an interesting specimen."

Leaving Lake Arenal, you'll head to the northwest and the Guanacaste, or gold coast region. "This is Costa Rica's cowboy country," Ronald continued. "The land is much flatter here, a combination of cattle ranches, dry tropical forest, and of course, beaches. It's much warmer here than around Arenal, close to 95 or 100 degrees. And the water is 80 degrees year-round." Riding along the coast, you can explore the different beaches. Playa Tamarindo is a world-renowned surfing spot. If you're curious about catching a wave,

OPPOSITE:
A tour of Costa Rica takes you from the cloud forests (shown here near the dormant volcano of Irazú) to the serene beaches of Guanacaste.

10

DESTINATION

some of the other beaches have consistent (though much smaller) waves that are ideal for beginners, and good instructors are available. Playa Conchal (which, as its name implies, has many shells) is a favorite kayaking venue, and there are several bays that offer wonderful snorkeling. "Come evening, you have some of Costa Rica's greatest sunsets," Ronald added. "It's as if the sky is on fire."

If you make it to Costa Rica and decide that you'd like a slightly more challenging ride, consider La Ruta de Los Conquistadores. This multiday mountain bike race traverses the American landmass some 240 miles (386 km) from the Pacific to the Caribbean, taking riders across five mountain ranges, with a total climb of 39,000 feet. The ride was inspired by a Costa Rican cyclist named Roman Urbina, who, having read of the twenty-year-long crossing of Costa Rica by the Spanish conquistadors Juan de Cavallón, Perafán de Rivera, and Juan Vásquez de Coronado, decided to replicate their passage on mountain bikes—generally in four days. "La Ruta attracts the world's best cyclists," Ronald added. "Chris Carmichael, Lance Armstrong's coach, came to do it the year of his fiftieth birthday, as he wanted a special physical and mental challenge to signify that milestone. I've done the race before. At the beginning on the Pacific side, I almost gave up from dehydration. When I reached the summit between the Pacific and the Caribbean side, I almost quit as I nearly got hypothermia from riding in the rain. It has not only extreme terrain, but also extreme conditions."

RONALD CALVO grew up in the province of Cartago, Costa Rica. He has worked at Universidad Latina de Costa Rica teaching geography and developmental planning and has lectured on geomorphology for the certification of tour guides at National Biodiversity Institute of Costa Rica and the National Learning Institute as well as for international students. Ronald also works as a freelance naturalist and adventure guide for DuVine Adventures, Lindblad/National Geographic Expeditions, Adventures by Disney, and Coasts & Mountains Adventures. A serious amateur racer, he's competed in the Costa Rica National Endurance Mountain Biking Championship, the Nevada State Championship, the Dick Evans Memorial, 112 miles around Oahu, Hawaii, and continues to enjoy exploring the roads around Cartago.

If You Go

▶ **Getting There:** Most international travelers to Costa Rica will fly into San José, Costa Rica, which is served by many carriers. Nature Air (800-235-9272; www.natureair.com) has service from Liberia (in Guanacaste) back to San José.

▶ **Best Time to Visit:** November to March is considered the "dry" season, though the tour described above can be taken throughout the year with the exception of September and October.

▶ **Guides/Outfitters:** Several outfitters lead bike-oriented tours in Costa Rica, including DuVine Adventures Bicycle Tours (888-396-5383; www.duvine.com).

▶ **Level of Difficulty:** The itinerary above involves four to five days of biking 20 to 25 miles (32 to 40 km) a day. It's rated moderate, given some off-road riding and warm temperatures.

▶ **Accommodations:** The following come well recommended: in San José, Hotel Grano de Oro (+506 2255 3322; www.granodeoro.com); near Arenal, Arenal Kioro Suites & Spa (+506 2479 1700; www.hotelarenalkioro.com); on the Guanacaste, Hotel La Posada (+506 2681 4318; www.laposadapinilla.com).

10

DESTINATION

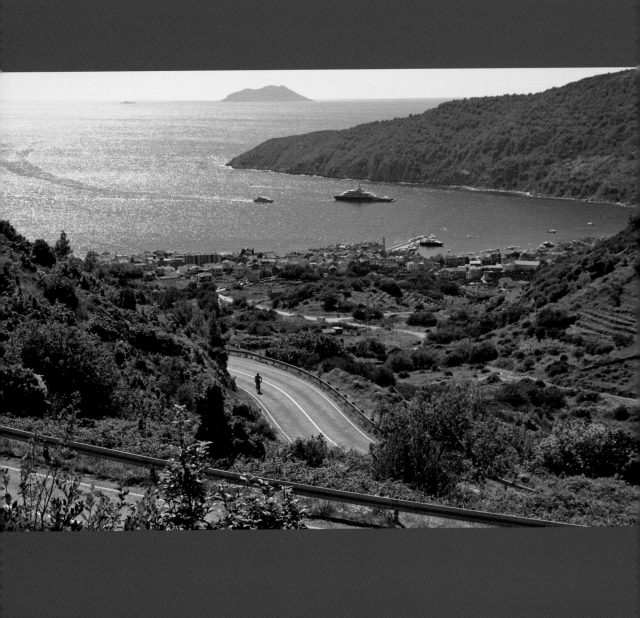

DALMATIAN COAST

RECOMMENDED BY **Chris Mark**

"I enjoy climbing," Chris Mark explained, "and get a kick out of watching the earth fall away below me. If there's water nearby to add color to this sense of accomplishment, all the better. The Dalmatian Coast of Croatia has hills and water in spades. And unlike a place like Connemara, Ireland, you can jump in and take a swim in all that lovely water that you pass. The biking is challenging, perhaps not for everybody, but the roads are well-paved, there's not much traffic, and each of the islands off the coast has its own character. Wherever you go, there's the smell of pines and sea. Up until fifty years ago, most of the villages on these islands were backwater fishing communities. By dint of that, they've been spared development."

Many travel business insiders consider Croatia a hidden gem, combining many of the best aspects of better-known southern European destinations—crystal-clear water, a mild climate, rich culture, and colorful cuisine—without the crowds. Croatia has a rich and incredibly complex history, a legacy that's reflected in the conflicts that have recently divided Yugoslavia. The turbulence that has dogged Croatia stems largely from its position at the nexus of central, southern, and eastern Europe, where Latin, Balkan, and Slavic cultures have freely intermingled. Croatia is across the Adriatic Sea from Italy (the city of Dubrovnik is at roughly the same latitude as Rome), and bordered by Hungary to the north, Slovenia to the northwest, and Montenegro to the southeast; Bosnia and Herzegovina cut into the center of the country, giving Croatia a horseshoe shape. The Croatian portion of the Dalmatian Coast spans from the border with Montenegro to the island of Rab in the northwest.

Chris's Dalmatian odyssey departed from Dubrovnik, a medieval walled city with a thoroughly modern vibe, a thriving café culture, and many fine restaurants. After a brief

OPPOSITE:
The island of Korcula, shown here, is one of your stops on a riding tour of the Dalmatian Coast.

tour of the city and a warm-up ride, Chris boarded a private *gulet* (the preferred sailing vessel in this region of the Adriatic) to begin his westward adventure. "It's wonderful to roll off the deck of the boat to do a 30- or 35-mile (50- or 60-km) ride on a coastal road across an island and have the boat waiting for you on the other side. You get connected right to the road, and you never have to backtrack over terrain you've already ridden."

The island-hopping itinerary Chris embarked on took him to Mljet, Korcula, Vis, and Hvar, before returning to the mainland at Split. Several rides stood out, including one on Mljet. "Mljet is not far from Dubrovnik, just south from the Pelješac Peninsula. Much of the island is preserved as a national park," Chris continued. "There aren't really towns in the park, just a few scattered settlements with restaurants and other basic services. The ride here is a point-to-point route—again, greatly facilitated by having a boat. It is one long road with a few side tracks. At one spot, you pass above an iconic white church on an island in a lake within the park—the Monastery of Saint Mary. [The original church was built in the late twelfth century by Benedictine monks from southern Italy.] Not long after the church, you begin climbing—a steady 8 or 9 percent grade. I'm not a grinder, so I stayed in a lower gear, trying to maintain a 95 cadence. Eventually you reach the spinal ridge of Mljet. It hasn't been cultivated for human use and reflects the land as it's been for many years—Mediterranean scrub pines, a few palm trees. Occasionally you break out of the trees and can see the ocean, other islands, even Dubrovnik in the distance. When you emerge from the forest, you're on a cliff, high above a bay and a small town, Prožurska Luka. At this point you turn off the main road, and there's a long sweeping downhill—you're riding the brakes most of the way. The road ends at the top of the town. From there, you either walk your bike or ride very carefully through the alleys. It's a spectacle of perfect Mediterraneanness. Once we returned to the boat, we could look back at the route we'd just taken."

The island that most impressed Chris was Vis. "Even by Croatian standards, Vis is off the beaten path. There's no daily ferry service from the mainland, so it doesn't get much tourist traffic. There are a lot of clichés in travel marketing about going back in time to untouched/unchanged places. Honestly, it's just not true. There are blue jeans and cell phones everywhere you go. But Vis is one of those places where you *almost* feel as though you're being transported to another time. As for the riding, there's a ring road that connects the two main towns—Vis Town and Komiza. You dip and dive along the cliff-side road, past olive groves and vineyards, with the blue Adriatic sparkling below.

"Beyond its uncrowded roads and Mediterranean ambiance, there's another great thing about bicycling in Croatia," Chris added. "You don't need notes. Most avid bikers are comfortable with a map in their back pocket. But when there's only one road, you don't need cue notes."

Croatia's cuisine bears some resemblance to southern Italian fare. There's a good deal of seafood (octopus is a favorite) as well as lamb. "The Croatians grow wonderful vegetables," Chris recalled. "What you'll get will depend on when you're there. Artichokes were in season during my visit. I came away pleasantly surprised by both the food and the wine. Some highly touted wines—both red and white—come from around the Pelješac Peninsula and Korcula. You can pleasantly drink the local wines, not feel like you're drinking them because you're obliged."

CHRIS MARK has worked in bicycle tourism on and off for more than twenty years, the past eight with Butterfield & Robinson, where he is responsible for the planning, research, and execution of its trips worldwide. Starting with a 6,000-mile European odyssey back in the day, Chris has pedaled roads from Latvia to Quebec to Japan's Noto Peninsula, though now family life limits him mostly to a 7-mile commute to work.

If You Go

▶ **Getting There:** Zagreb is served by many airlines, including Air France, British Airways, and KLM via Amsterdam, Frankfurt, and other European cities. From Zagreb, Croatia Airlines (www.croatiaairlines.hr) provides service to either Dubrovnik or Split.

▶ **Best Time to Visit:** Most visitors prefer to bike from late spring through early fall.

▶ **Guides/Outfitters:** Several outfitters lead trips in Croatia, including Butterfield & Robinson (866-551-9090; www.butterfield.com).

▶ **Level of Difficulty:** The trip above involves six days of riding. Though distances are short (none more than 25 miles [40 km]), terrain is hilly, thus the ride is rated moderate to difficult.

▶ **Onshore Accommodations:** The Croatian National Tourist Board (+385 4699 333; www.croatia.hr) lists lodging options all along the Dalmatian Coast.

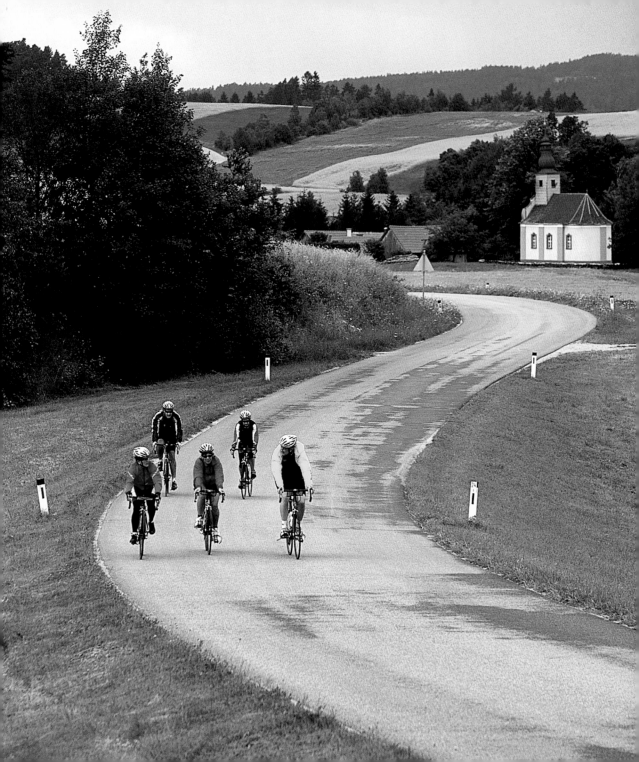

PRAGUE TO VIENNA

RECOMMENDED BY **Angela Horvath Burke**

The region along the border of the Czech Republic and Austria—the heart of Bohemia—has special resonance for Angela Horvath Burke. "The very first riding trip I was hired to guide on was Prague to Vienna," she began, "and I've done it about twenty times since. I've lived in Prague and Germany, have relatives in the region, and can speak both Czech and German." Those riders with less immediate ties to the region will find many reasons to embrace it as well, from ice-cold Budvar and enchanting Rieslings to medieval villages, baroque abbeys, and the storybook landscapes of the Danube River valley. (One small note: Though the trip is billed Prague to Vienna, riding starts south of the Czech capital and ends north of Vienna. "People get to enjoy Prague and Vienna on their own," Angela added. "It's a little too busy to ride comfortably in these cities.")

After a morning shuttle from Prague, your first stop is the Budweiser Budvar Brewery—the original Budweiser, dating back to the late 1700s. "Beer is quite important to the Czech people," Angela continued. "They drink 1.5 liters (48 oz) of beer per day, more per capita than any other country. Budvar lager tastes nothing like Anheuser-Busch products. It's a lager, but has a slightly sweeter taste, almost like a Weiss beer. We get a private tour of the brewery; this immersion in a key part of Czech culture sets the tone of how the trip will roll." The shuttle drops riders off in the medieval city of Český Krumlov, which has been aggressively preserved for more than one hundred years. (The translation of *Krumlov* is "crooked meadow," as the city wraps around the Vltava River.) "We're based here for a few days, and take some moderate rides through farmland and rolling hills outside the city, terrain that's not unlike Wisconsin. These rides give you an insight into how rural Czech people live. There's also the option of paddling down the Vltava. Of course, you get a chance to sample Czech cuisine. Standard fare is pretty meat-focused,

OPPOSITE:

The ride from Prague to Vienna highlights rural life in central Europe.

65

with lots of pork, boar, and beef, as well as hearty dumpling-style dishes. During a walking tour of the town, I also like to sample the street food. A favorite is dough that's roasted over open coals and then dipped in cinnamon or almonds."

On day three, riders cross from the Czech Republic into Austria, and the tour kicks into a lower gear—literally. "The Czech border is ringed by mountains, so there are some good challenges for your legs as we cross the border. The weather in the southern Czech Republic can often be cool and rainy, the dreary image North Americans might have of central Europe. But when we cross the border into Austria, the sun seems to always come out. In just over a quarter mile (half a kilometer), the infrastructure changes dramatically. The roads are much smoother, the flower boxes are brighter, there's no chipped paint on the houses. Despite their geographic proximity, Austria and the Czech Republic couldn't be more different. I think of this as our 'Hills Are Alive' day—the scenery is stunningly beautiful in a *Sound of Music* way. We stay at Schlosshotel Rosenau, which was established as a castle in the late 1500s. The approach to the hotel is quite dramatic, as you're riding through the countryside and suddenly there's this great baroque castle."

The next day, you'll continue along the quiet roads of northern Austria's Waldviertel region, where most traffic is limited to farmers and other cyclists. "Though we've moved beyond the border region, there's still lots of good climbing," Angela continued. "This is the peak of the riding for serious bikers. The lunch stop is perhaps the best of the trip, a tiny family-run restaurant called Gasthof Schindler that serves the best Wiener schnitzel and apple strudel. (Though Austrian cuisine is a bit lighter and more refined than Czech fare, it's still meat-oriented.) I tell fellow riders that they'll have to climb a bit to get to lunch, but not to worry about chowing down on fried pork, as it's downhill from here into the Danube River valley and the Wachau region. You pass through little villages that might have two hundred residents, a little butcher shop, and a bakery. Finally, we reach the village of Dürnstein. In Dürnstein, I love to dine at least one night in one of the rustic wine taverns—*Heurigen*, in German—which are usually associated with a nearby vineyard. Though beer is still part of the culture here, this is first and foremost white wine country, with a host of crisp Rieslings and Gewürztraminers. At the Alter Klosterkeller, they put down a smorgasbord of freshly cut horseradish, fifteen types of cheese, and twenty styles of prosciutto. All is washed down with local wines before the main meat course is served. If it's a nice evening, we might sit out in the vineyard. You can watch the Danube flow by, and even hear the water."

For Angela, the fifth day of the tour—the ride to the monastery at Melk and back to Dürnstein—is perhaps the world's most pleasurable ride. "The ride—part of it on the Passau bike trail that goes to Vienna—rolls along the Danube, through vineyard after vineyard, past apple orchards," she enthused. "It's mostly flat, and the sun is at your back; it's almost always sunny and temperate. Everything scopes upward on either side as you ride along, and the hills are dotted with castles from the thirteenth and fourteenth centuries. You can stop and grab an apple or plum or some grapes right from the tree or vine. In Melk, you can tour Stift Melk, a Benedictine abbey that was built in the early 1700s. It's a celebrated example of baroque design. On the way back to Dürnstein, the sun is again at your back, and you can stop in the towns along the way to sample local wines. In so many ways, it's just a perfect place to ride your bike."

ANGELA HORVATH BURKE has been employed with Trek Travel for more than five years. She started out as a guide, working trips like Prague to Vienna, Tuscany, California Wine Country, and others. She now works at the home office in Madison, Wisconsin, doing sales outreach. She enjoys cycling, traveling, and spending time at home with her growing family.

If You Go

▶ **Getting There:** Most visitors will fly into Prague at the ride's beginning and fly out of Vienna at the ride's conclusion. Both cities are served by many international carriers.

▶ **Best Time to Visit:** Late spring to early fall provides the most reliable weather.

▶ **Guides/Outfitters:** A number of companies lead bike tours of this region, including Trek Travel (866-464-8735; www.trektravel.com). Do-it-yourselfers might visit the Friends of Czech Greenways website (www.pragueviennagreenways.org).

▶ **Level of Difficulty:** The trip above entails six days of riding an average 25 miles (40 km) per day; it's rated moderate.

▶ **Accommodations:** On their more luxurious itinerary, Trek guides stop at Hotel Růže (+420 380 772 100; www.hotelruze.cz) in Český Krumlov, Schlosshotel Rosenau in Zwettl (+432 822 582 210; www.schlosshotel.rosenau.at), and Hotel Schloss Dürnstein (+432 711 212; www.schloss.at).

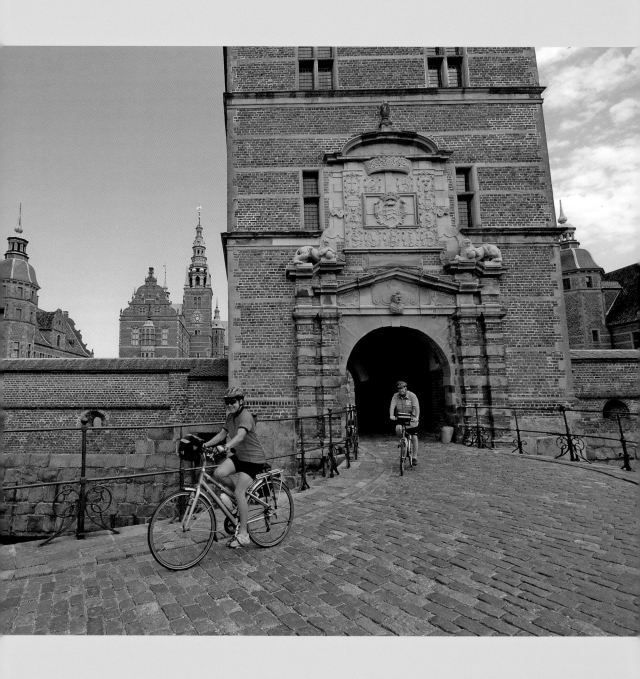

DANISH ISLES

RECOMMENDED BY **Ron van Dijk**

When Americans think of European bike touring vacations, Denmark is generally way down the list if it's on the list at all. Ron van Dijk thinks that Scandinavia's southernmost nation deserves more attention from the cycling community.

"I believe Denmark is one of the great countries for biking," Ron explained. "First, biking is a huge part of Danish culture. All the locals travel by bike, especially when they go on vacation. You'll come upon whole families going by bike. The dad might be pulling a child along while mom has toddlers on special bikes with little platforms in front. When you bike around Denmark, you're like one of the locals, and that makes for a special experience. The infrastructure seems as if it were custom-made for cyclists. There are bike paths everywhere, special bike lanes and traffic lights in the more urban areas, plus there are towns every 3 miles (5 km) or so, even in the rural areas. When I first visited in 1987, I was expecting the land to be flat; instead, the topography—especially along the islands to the east—was marked by undulating hills. There are new vistas after each hill, and you're never far from the water—be it the Øresund (the narrow strait that separates the Danish island of Zealand from Sweden) or the many lakes that dot the islands. For me, it's always wonderful to have water nearby as you ride. The houses in the countryside—many half-timbered, with thatched roofs, the inspiration for what's known in England as Tudor style—are very well kept. They give you a feeling of old Europe."

Denmark, which is tucked between Germany to the south and Sweden and Norway to the north, is divided between Jutland (the mainland, which "juts" into the North Sea) and more than four hundred islands that dot the waters between Jutland and southern Sweden. Ron likes to focus his riding along the islands of Zealand, Funen, and Aerø, beginning in Copenhagen. "On many of the rides I lead, we tend to avoid urban traffic,

OPPOSITE:
Cyclists roll
through the
Frederiksborg
Slot near the
former royal
castle in Hillerød.

DESTINATION

13

but Copenhagen is so bike-friendly, I don't mind riding here," he said. "Some of the bike lanes are as wide as car lanes." Copenhagen may be known in some circles for its laissez-faire attitudes toward—um—casual interpersonal relationships, though it's increasingly recognized for its aggressive pro-bike policies and the way its citizenry has embraced bike commuting. The numbers tell all: Out of 1.2 million residents, roughly 500,000 commuters choose to bike to work each day!

"From Copenhagen, we make our way along the Øresund, on a stretch known as the Danish Riviera," Ron continued. "This is where many of Copenhagen's well-to-do have retired or keep second homes. The houses are lovely, and the bike paths are close to the sea. I love to visit the Louisiana Museum of Modern Art, which is along this stretch. It's built right on the water, and light reflecting off the Øresund comes in the windows. I also find the Karen Blixen Museum (the home of the Danish author of *Out of Africa,* among other titles) inspiring." Your education in things Danish continues as you ride to Helsingør, which readers of Shakespeare might remember as *Elsinore,* home of a certain famously unsettled prince. There's a library stack's worth of doctoral theses concerning whether there was in fact a historical Hamlet, and if there was, how much his story influenced the Bard. Hamlet or not, Helsingør *is* the site of the royal castle of Kronborg, parts of which date back to the late sixteenth century. The structure is a wonderful example of Renaissance architecture, and its strategic location gave Denmark a perfect outpost to monitor potential interlopers at the narrowest point of the Øresund. If visitors wish, they can pop over to Sweden by ferry for dinner in less than twenty minutes.

From Helsingør and the island of Zealand, the tour transfers to the island of Funen, with a stop in the town of Roskilde at the Viking Ship Museum and the Roskilde Cathedral. "The Vikings sank a number of ships near Roskilde in what seems to have been a ritual," Ron continued. "The crafts, which date back to the ninth and tenth centuries, are very well preserved. You get a great sense of the Vikings' skill as boatbuilders. Having the fastest ships enabled them to be successful raiders. The cathedral is of great significance to the Danes, as all of Denmark's kings and queens since the ninth century are buried here. It would be a great location for a horror movie, with all the graves!"

The next day, you'll hop a ferry and explore Aerø Island. "This island has splendid coastal scenery, with picturesque fishing villages," Ron enthused. "Some of the best examples of half-timbered houses are here. They're built by setting up the frame of wooden beams and filling in the rest of the space with bricks or straw. Before returning to

Copenhagen, I like to stop at the Hans Christian Andersen Museum, which does an excellent job of portraying his fairy tales. The Ugly Duckling tale is said to be based on him.

"When I reflect on my rides along the Danish Isles, I always come back to the image of the many happy Danish families cycling, the radiant smiles on their faces, and all that blond hair. The last time I did the trip, some of my guests commented that Denmark seemed to have the happiest people they'd seen anywhere in the world. Maybe it's because of the government's generous social programs. In Denmark, people don't seem to mind paying taxes; they believe their money comes back to them."

RON VAN DIJK got his start in the biking/travel business in 1983, and is proud to say he hasn't stopped pedaling since. Born and raised in Holland, Ron has spent most of his life in the Netherlands, Germany, and France. By the time he was twenty-one, he had explored a good portion of Europe and was fluent in Dutch, German, French, and English. Since then he has learned Spanish and Italian. Without a language barrier, Ron has access to people, places, and a true insider's perspective, which he shares with every guest. He is now director of European operations for Austin-Lehman Adventures.

If You Go

▶ **Getting There:** Most fly into Copenhagen, which is served by many major carriers.

▶ **Best Time to Visit:** June may be the best month for a trip, though July through September also offer consistent weather, albeit with more crowds.

▶ **Guides/Outfitters:** A number of outfitters lead bike trips around Denmark, including Austin-Lehman Adventures (800-575-1540; www.austinlehman.com).

▶ **Level of Difficulty:** This tour entails six days of riding, with an average of 25 miles (40 km) a day. It's rated easy to moderate.

▶ **Accommodations:** Ron recommends the following lodging options for the route described above: Hotel Phoenix Copenhagen (+45 3395 9500; www.phoenixcopenhagen .com), Hotel Marienlyst (+45 4921 4000; www.marienlyst.dk/uk.html), Hotel Svendborg (+45 6221 1700; www.hotel-svendborg.dk), and Hotel Faaborg Fjord (+45 6261 1010; www.hotelfaaborgfjord.dk).

13

DESTINATION

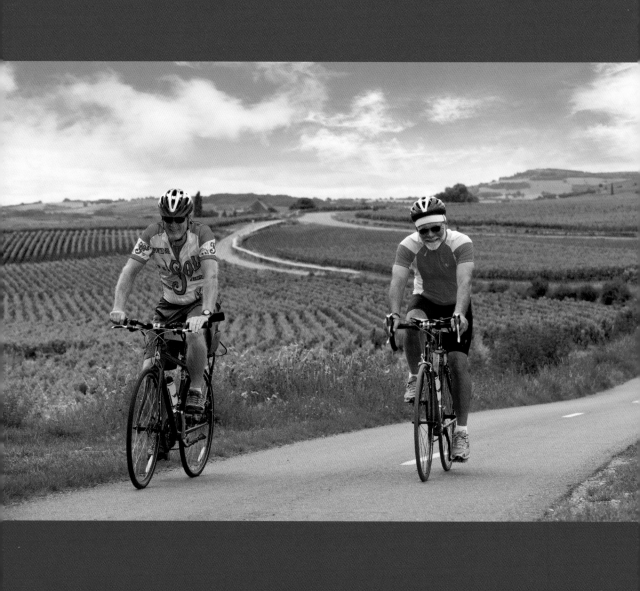

BURGUNDY

RECOMMENDED BY **George Butterfield**

"Before I first visited Burgundy and the walled city of Beaune in the early 1980s, it was typical for traveling bicyclists to stay in youth hostels," George Butterfield led off. "About this time, we had the idea of pairing wonderful places to stay with great places to bike. Why shouldn't cyclists stay in good hotels? When we discovered Beaune, I fell in love. I think it's the greatest biking destination in the world—the rides, the red wines, the beauty and authenticity of the town, a place where real people live and make wine, the great elixir of life. I could go riding every day for a month and my route would never be the same. When I come down off the hills and drift into Beaune, I feel like I've been in heaven. Butterfield & Robinson made it headquarters for our European operations not long after my first visit. It was like they built the city just for us—how thoughtful!"

The Burgundy (or *Bourgogne* in French) region rests in eastern France; the area's capital, Dijon, is a two-hour high-speed train ride from Paris. The region's documented wine history goes back nearly two millennia; Clos de Vougeot, the oldest and one of the largest vineyards currently operating in Burgundy, was established by monks in 1115. The Côte d'Or—a limestone escarpment that runs through the heart of Bourgogne—is the foundation of the *terroir* that has bred some of the world's finest wines. This is primarily Pinot Noir and Chardonnay country, though several other grapes (including Aligoté and Gamay) are also grown. "Burgundian wines are known for their purity; reds are made exclusively from Pinot Noir grapes, whites entirely from Chardonnays," said David Butterfield, son of George and owner of Beaune-based Butterfield Wines. "In Bordeaux, winemakers eagerly blend different varietals together, a process considered just short of blasphemy in Burgundy. To my palate, the wines of Burgundy are soft, elegant, and unquestionably complex."

OPPOSITE:
Cycling out of Beaune, you'll pass some of the world's most celebrated vineyards.

While Dijon may be the region's administrative hub, Beaune is considered Burgundy's wine capital. With many battlements and ramparts from medieval times (and earlier) still intact, Beaune seems as braced to repel the marauding onslaught of cheap varietals from upstarts abroad as it once was to stave off unfriendly visitors. But it certainly has its charms. As Bruce Schoenfeld wrote of Beaune in the December 2010 issue of *Travel & Leisure,*

> Buildings in stone and earth tones surround the main square, which is fashioned as precisely as a movie set. Shops selling mundane items are impossibly beautiful. It's an idealized rendering of a French medieval town adapted for modern existence. History suffuses the streets, to such an extent that I've always wondered if Beaune's crowded past—full of Romans and dukes, cardinals and kings—leaves room for daily life.

The village is home to Hospices de Beaune, a hospital for the indigent established in 1443. More important for our purposes, Beaune is a splendid point of departure for a panoply of rides on the thousands of miles of quiet, paved roads that slice through the adjoining countryside. George described one favorite: "It takes you only about four to five minutes to bike out of Beaune, and I love to head south to Pommard. As you climb slowly through the vines, you'll encounter a few other cyclists and perhaps some tractors, but little else. You'll pass a number of different appellations; with luck, one of your companions will be able to explain them as you pause to take everything in. Soon you'll leave the vines as you begin the climb to St. Romain, an ancient city with a castle that dates back to the 1100s. It's one of the great climbs in the region, and when you have the chance to look down over the vines from where you've come, you think, 'I've had a most magnificent climb.' Then you ride up to Orches, a hidden little town. No one says a word when we get to Orches, a magical place where the great wines grow.

"From Orches, we begin to head back to Beaune, via the picturesque village of La Rochepot. The castle here—once the home of the Dukes of Burgundy—is quite well preserved. We're a bit outside of the wine country here, but soon we'll return. From La Rochepot, we proceed to Bâtard-Montrachet. Anyone who doesn't bow down in reverence to Bâtard-Montrachet—home of one of the world's great white wines—is crazy. A little sip of wine at 11 a.m. is very satisfying. After paying your respects, you come back into the villages. You'd stop and have a bit of lunch, perhaps in Pommard, and continue on. If it were me leading the ride, we'd next stop in Meursault at my son David's winery, and have a tasting of Chardonnay out of the barrel. From there, we'd glide back to Beaune. The ride is five or six hours, with fine wines, restaurants, and good climbs. It's less than 30 miles (50 km). If I had only one ride to do in a lifetime, this would be it."

With nearly thirty years of riding in Burgundy—and now, a home in Beaune—George Butterfield has a trunkload of memories from the esteemed wine region. "I recall a certain night in July. There was a full moon. My companions and I had dinner at Le Chassagne in Chassagne-Montrachet. Le Chassagne has what may be the finest Burgundy collection anywhere. Sometimes you have too much wine, but this night we were restrained, consuming just two or three glasses over dinner. I'll always remember drifting back into Beaune in the full moonlight, with no pedaling and not a word among us. Nothing needed to be said."

GEORGE BUTTERFIELD organized a student biking trip in France in 1966 with his wife, Martha, and her brother, Sidney Robinson. That pioneering venture evolved into Butterfield & Robinson, the world's premier luxury active travel company. Still at it after all these years, George continues to serve as B&R's spiritual leader, resident travel sage, voyageur extraordinaire, and CEO of all things slow. He is always on the hunt for new and interesting places to explore, but his favorite trip is always the one he's taking next.

If You Go

▶ **Getting There:** International visitors will generally fly into Paris and take a high-speed train to Dijon, launching point for many Burgundy sojourns.

▶ **Best Time to Visit:** Most riders prefer to visit Burgundy in May through October.

▶ **Guides/Outfitters:** Outfitters leading trips around Burgundy include Butterfield & Robinson (866-551-9090; www.butterfield.com) and VBT (800-245-3868; www.vbt.com).

▶ **Level of Difficulty**: The itinerary above includes five days of riding, covering between 17 and 27 miles (27 and 44 km) a day. It's rated moderate.

▶ **Accommodations:** A favorite resting place in Beaune is L'Hôtel de Beaune (+33 0 3 80 25 94 14; www.lhoteldebeaune.com). In Chambolle-Musigny, George likes Château André Ziltener (+33 0 3 80 62 41 62; www.chateau-ziltener.com) and in La Bussière-sur-Ouche, Abbaye de la Bussière, (+33 0 3 80 49 02 29; www.abbayedelabussiere.fr).

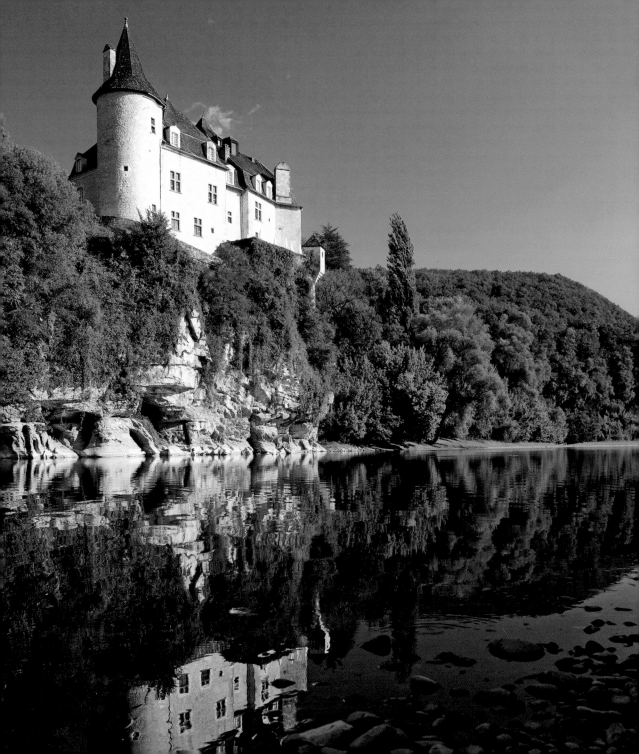

DORDOGNE

RECOMMENDED BY **Renée Krysko**

You traverse roller-coaster hills, swooping up and down through a canopy of trees. As you wind around a corner, a medieval castle flashes into view. Navigate another curve and another castle appears, perched high above a gently flowing river. Paleolithic art beckons once you step out of the saddle . . . as does duck magret and other local delicacies.

You're in the Dordogne, one of Renée Krysko's favorite places to ride a bike. "The Dordogne is a fascinating area on so many levels, and all the rides showcase the region's colorful aspects," she began. "Cruising along the river, you'll see castles towering over you for miles and miles. It's like you've gone back into medieval times. From the strategic placement of fortresses and the reputation of its wines, to the evolution of both the French and English languages, the region and its culture was very much shaped by the Hundred Years War that was fought by the French and English. It's a place that has kept much of its authenticity. And with fewer North American tourists than other sites in France, Americans will feel like they are truly in a unique place. The constantly hilly terrain will get your heartbeat up—it's 100 meters up, then down, 75 meters up, then down, 200 meters up, then down. If you'd like, you can opt to cycle along the river."

Dordogne is situated in the southwest of France, between the Loire Valley and the Pyrenees. It takes its name from the river that flows through the region to the Atlantic. "There's a story, perhaps apocryphal," Renée continued, "that during the Hundred Years War, people in the Dordogne would transport a local wine called Cahors (a blend made up primarily of Malbec grapes and produced in and around the village of Cahors) to Bordeaux for export to other parts of France and England. It's said that Bordeaux residents would dump the wine in the river and export their own wines instead, helping to assure that it was Bordeaux wines that gained a reputation."

OPPOSITE:

Perched above the Dordogne River, Château de la Treyne is a favorite stopover for many cyclists.

After gathering in the city of Bergerac, you'll cross the river to the village of Monbazillac, and your ride will begin—perhaps after a sample of the sweet white wine that's created here. A peaceful ride through vineyards, farmland, and quaint villages takes you to the village of Trémolat. "In Trémolat, I like to stay at Le Vieux Logis," Renée said. "The property has been in the same family for more than four hundred years. Lodging is in an old farmhouse. Though it's a four-star hotel and quite sumptuous, you don't feel as though you can't touch anything. There's a lovely pool and gardens, so refreshing after a ride. The restaurant here is Michelin-starred. I particularly remember a dessert they often serve, a chocolate lava cake. Rich dark chocolate pours out from the middle as your fork penetrates the cake. The quality of the chocolate is divine, and it's augmented with a raspberry or lavender coulis."

A special treat awaits when you roll out of Trémolat, cross the Dordogne once again, and arrive at Les Eyzies-sur-Tayac—the prehistoric cave paintings of Font de Gaume. "The morning's ride is quite hilly on tree-shaded roller-coaster roads," Renée described. "After a stop at a farmers' market in the village of Le Bugue and a picnic lunch in Les Eyzies, we take a private tour of the caves (which archaeologists and art historians consider the best example of polychrome painting other than those at Lascaux, which are now closed to the public). Our private guide—a gentleman named Bart—ties in the evolution of the people of the Magdalénien period and discusses the possible meaning of this site and the art found inside. He theorizes that with the development of the frontal lobe, humans became separate from nature. And that perhaps this site embodies our early notions of religion, art, and science and our attempt to reconnect to nature." The paintings—more than two hundred in all—include eighty bison, forty horses, and some twenty mammoths; they date back to 14000 BC. "From the stunning ride and the taste of small village life, to the tour of Font-de-Gaume," Renée added, "it's a once-in-a-lifetime kind of experience."

The next stop as you ride through Dordogne is Sarlat; in Renée's opinion, it is the most unbelievable village in all of France. "Some years back, the French government embarked on a preservation/beautification project of several historic sites, including Sarlat. They cleaned up the stone buildings, installed gas lanterns to illuminate the town at night, among other improvements. Today, the town has a splendid medieval feeling. If you happen to visit on a Saturday, you must go to the market. It is the best market in France. As you wander the narrow lanes, there are stalls with ducks hanging upside down, cheesemongers, vendors selling foie gras and fresh flowers, and buskers playing music. You feel like you've traveled through time. Food is very important to the people in Dordogne, and they're very selective about what they eat. You see that passion in the market." The Dordogne River was the front line of the Hundred Years War in the fourteenth and fifteenth century. During your stay in Sarlat, you'll have the chance to glide the river by canoe, taking in the castles and fortresses along the Dordogne much as the soldiers did. You may wish to visit one of the formidable castles—Château de Beynac, which was built atop a limestone cliff above the river in the twelfth century, and has been used as the site for several movies. "The Dordogne," Renée concluded, "is the birthplace of what is the best of France—the food, the culture, the architecture, the history. I can't wait to return."

RENÉE KRYSKO has been employed with Trek Travel for more than eight years. She started as a guide, working trips like Provence, the Tour de France, Classic Climbs of the Dolomites, Dordogne, and others. She then moved on to working on trip design in France and Canada, as well as on marketing and guide training. She enjoys cycling, traveling (obviously), dancing, and spending time playing outside in the Rocky Mountains of Canada.

If You Go

▶ **Getting There:** International visitors will generally fly into Paris and take a high-speed train to Bergerac, the point of departure for Renée's itinerary.

▶ **Best Time to Visit:** May through October provides the best riding conditions.

▶ **Guides/Outfitters:** A number of outfitters lead bike trips around the Dordogne region, including Trek Travel (866-464-8735; www.trektravel.com).

▶ **Level of Difficulty:** The itinerary above has five days of riding, with an average of 35 miles (56 km) per day. It's rated moderate.

▶ **Accommodations:** For the route described above, Trek recommends the following hotels: in Trémolat, Le Vieux Logis (+33 0 5 53 22 80 06; www.vieux-logis.com); in Sarlat, Hôtel Clos la Boétie (+33 0 5 53 29 44 18; www.closlaboetie-sarlat.com); and Château de la Treyne (+33 5 65 27 60 60; www.chateaudelatreyne.com).

DESTINATION 15

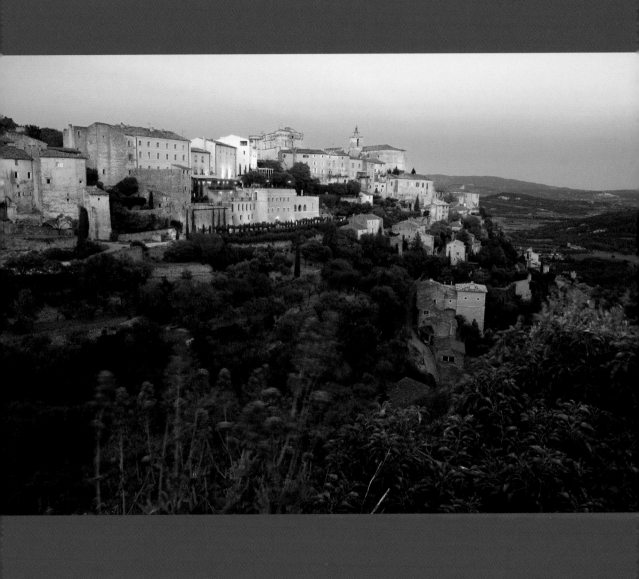

PROVENCE

RECOMMENDED BY **Jeneen Sutherland**

Any cyclist who's read Peter Mayles's *A Year in Provence* has likely pondered the prospect of one day visiting this region in the south of France. No matter how much reading you've done, though, it's difficult to prepare for the onslaught Provence launches upon your senses. The light, thick and rich, bounces off every surface. The smell of the air, redolent with spices from the profusion of rosemary, thyme, fennel, and lavender growing wild, offers up a delicious aroma. And finally, there are the people. Locals identify with their Provençal heritage and celebrate a way of life that stands apart from the rest of France. Biking around the region lets you match that regional pace to better appreciate it.

"When you poke around on your bike in Provence and take the time to cruise through the middle of the little towns—linger in the markets, lunch at local bistros—you get a taste of the authentic Provence," Jeneen Sutherland said. "And to make things even better, the region offers some of the finest cycling you can hope for. You can still find many quiet, tiny roads that are a dream to cycle on. There's just the right amount of hills to keep you honest, but if you've had a tough climb, there's an easy downhill waiting for you. I guided in Provence fifteen times, and I never tired of it. Between zipping up and down from one fairy-tale village to another on the hilltops of the Luberon Valley and riding among the plentiful Roman ruins, you could easily go 50 or 60 miles (80 to 100 km) each day and never repeat yourself. Provence is ever-changing: In spring, everything is in bloom, and you're riding by fields of bright red poppies. In the fall, the vineyards are a riot of color. And in late June and early July, it's lavender season. The postcards you see are no joke. In the town of Sault, the hillsides are festooned in lavender. When you ride the descent from Gorges de la Nesque and come into the flats, lavender is everywhere—you feel like it's being massaged into your temples!"

OPPOSITE:
The stunning hill town of Gordes.

There are many moments to be cherished as you ride through Provence. Near the town of Collias, the greens of the rolling vineyards and Technicolor yellow of the stands of sunflowers are eventually broken by the monolithic Pont du Gard, a Roman aqueduct built more than two thousand years ago to carry water some 30 miles (48 km) to the town of Nîmes; it's considered one of the Roman empire's most enduring engineering achievements. You may come upon villagers convening for a game of *boules* (similar to lawn bowling) and even join in, or enjoy a refreshing pastis, an anise-flavored liqueur served cold that's usually diluted with water until it assumes a pale yellow hue.

Your thoughts will sooner or later wander to food. Mealtimes showcase Provence at its very finest. "The cuisine is earthy, simple," Jeneen continued, "not as rich and heavy as the food in northern France. Much of what's eaten might be called peasant food—ratatouille, bouillabaisse, chèvre with herbs or flowers. The plentitude of the local markets is overwhelming! Each little town has its specialty. And there are many great, small mom-and-pop wineries everywhere you turn." Châteauneuf-du-Pape (a blend of predominately Grenache grapes) is one favorite; Bandols, one of the unsung wines of France, are also special, with hints of spice and effervescence.

For many cyclists visiting Provence, the greatest challenge may be squeezing into the biking shorts you arrived in after so much good food and wine. For the serious, perhaps even masochistic rider, there's Mont Ventoux, the luminous white limestone spire that towers a mile above the surrounding countryside. Mont Ventoux—as prominent and jarring a landmass as Wyoming's Devils Tower—has figured prominently in a number of Tour de France races; the grueling climb contributed to the death of British cyclist Tom Simpson in the 1967 tour. "I almost always make a point to climb Mont Ventoux when I'm cycling around Provence," Jeneen said, "usually before the main trip begins. I still remember the very first time. One of my fellow guides and I had made a plan to do the ride early in the morning from our inn in Bédoin. We were supposed to meet at 6 a.m. When I got up at 5:30, it was pouring down rain. I was so psyched about doing the ride, I decided I'd go for it, even though my friend had begged off.

"I'd read about the climb and kind of knew what to expect: 5,250 feet (1,600 meters) of climbing over 13 miles (22 km), with some grades of more than 10 percent, and an average grade of 7 or 8 percent. As I began the climb out of the valley, looking out over the vineyards, the rain continued to pour down, leaking through my cycling glasses. As I rode through the pine forests in the lower reaches of Mont Ventoux, I felt like I could smell the rain. I entered a meditative state over the course of the two hours it took me to reach the top. Coming out of the pine forest, you enter into this lunar-like landscape. At this point, I rose above the clouds, and it was sunny and clear. I'm not a very spiritual person, but I felt like I was having an out-of-body experience. When I reached the panoramic marker, I was totally moved. It was very evident why this climb can break some riders, and at the same time, it's clear why it's considered such an amazing experience. During the Tour de France, people camp out on the side of the road a week in advance. To do the ride during the tour is awesome. Mont Ventoux can be superpainful, but it's certainly a ride serious cyclists must do before they die."

JENEEN SUTHERLAND is the director of bespoke travel for Butterfield & Robinson. She took a break from her designing job to guide for B&R ten years ago and never looked back! Since joining B&R, she has traveled all over the world as a regional director, trip manager, and now director of bespoke. Jeneen lives in Vancouver with her husband (a B&R boy himself) and their two active children. Her favorite thing to do when not planning trips? Playing with her kids by the ocean or cycling in the mountains by her home.

If You Go

▶ **Getting There:** Trips will begin in Avignon, which can be reached via train from Paris.
▶ **Best Time to Visit:** Mid-May through mid-October, though July and August may be a bit warm for some cyclists.
▶ **Guides/Outfitters:** Most international bike touring outfits lead trips to Provence, including Butterfield & Robinson (866-551-9090; www.butterfield.com).
▶ **Level of Difficulty:** The trip above entails five days of riding with daily distances averaging 31 miles (50 km). It's rated moderate, though the climb of Mont Ventoux is quite challenging.
▶ **Accommodations:** A few inns that Jeneen and Butterfield & Robinson recommend are Le Coquillade (+33 0 4 90 74 71 71; www.coquillade.fr) and La Bastide de Marie (+33 0 4 50 63 20; http://en.labastidedemarie.com) in Luberon, Le Hameau des Baux (+33 0 4 90 54 10 30; www.hameaudesbaux.com/uk) in Paradou, and Château de Mazan (+33 4 90 69 62 61; www.chateaudemazan.com/uk) in Mazan.

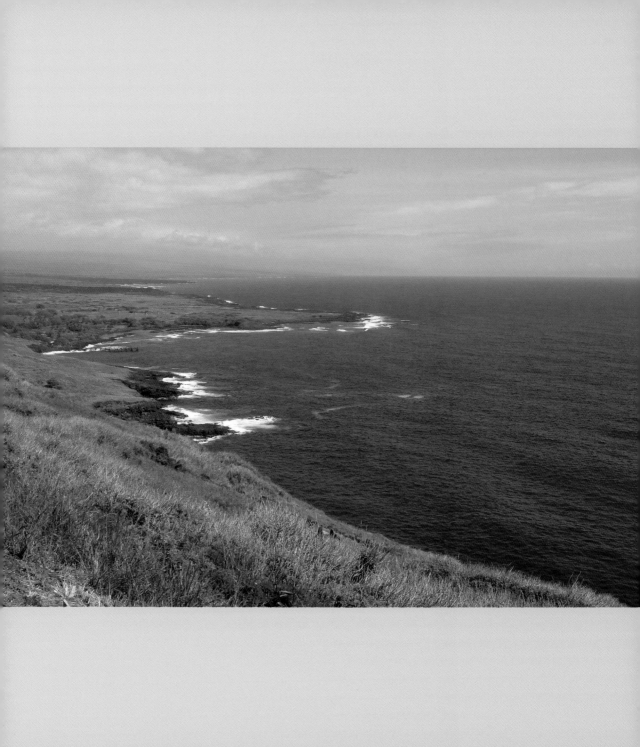

BIG ISLAND

RECOMMENDED BY **Julie Robinson**

The Big Island of Hawaii offers cyclists one of nature's most impressive smorgasbords: a frequently snowcapped mountain, active volcanoes gurgling magma into the Pacific, and eleven of the world's thirteen climate zones encompassing a staggeringly diverse ecosystem. Add in a panoply of isolated beaches, cultural landmarks that tell the story of humankind's earliest endeavors in Hawaii, and top it all off with a well-paved coastal road that connects everything, and you have the makings of an epic ride.

"I'd been to the Hawaiian islands a few times before," Julie Robinson said, "but I was shocked at how different the Big Island was from Maui and Oahu. The stage is set when you land, as the airport is on a lava field. It's amazing to think that the island is still growing! As you ride clockwise from north to south, the island slowly unfolds and tells its own story, from the stark transitions between landscapes to the history of King Kamehameha. This is a different Hawaii from the one many of us are sold, and biking the coastline over a week takes you to places that many visitors don't get to see."

Julie's ride began in Waimea at Parker Ranch, in what's come to be called the Big Island's cowboy country. "It's all cacti, chickens, and cows in a fairly dry environment," she continued. "The road heads south along the island's east side, so you start with a fairly easy ride through farmlands. At one point you go up a hill and around a corner and *bam!*, you're in the jungle. You can smell the ginger and hibiscus in the air. After a great downhill past the town of Honokaa, you reach the overlook above Waipio Valley, the birthplace of King Kamehameha. The cliffs, blanketed in tropical foliage, plunge down more than 1,000 feet. It's a sacred place for Hawaiians, and you feel shrouded in the mists of history. The rest of the ride to Hilo goes past coconut and banana plantations, with mountains on your right and the Pacific on your left. The trees smell wonderful."

OPPOSITE:
The coast as you roll toward Hawi, the finishing point of your circumnavigation of the Big Island.

The second day of the ride is Julie's favorite of the trip, taking you along the east side of Hawaii to Kilauea Crater, through the seldom-visited-by-tourists district of Pahoa. There's very little traffic on this two-lane road on Wednesdays," Julie continued. "You start out riding through forests of eucalyptus, with peekaboo glimpses of the sparkling blue ocean now and then. The road comes out right at the coast, and for 5 or 6 miles (8 or 9 km), the eucalyptus give way to banyans. Some of these trees are more than one hundred years old, and they lace over the road. It's a magical stretch. I love to stop at a small park—Isaac Hale Beach Park—that comes up soon after. The park has a hot pool (Pohoiki Warm Springs) that sits in a lava sink and is fed by a volcanic spring; it's like a hot tub for two hundred people, surrounded by palms. There's a breakwater that keeps the ocean out, but the spray drifts over the edge. We stop that evening at Kilauea Lodge, which is adjacent to Volcanoes National Park. Kilauea is one of the world's most active volcanoes. If nature is cooperating, you can head into the park after dinner and watch molten lava flow into the sea, like a glowing red river."

Many riders will choose to lay over at Kilauea for a day to explore the park. One option is to do the 6-mile (9.5 km) Kilauea Crater hike; another is to cycle around Kilauea's rim. For those eager for more miles, there's the ride to Mauna Loa, the world's largest volcano. "It's a long ride, not for everyone," Julie opined, "but once you're up there, it's a stellar view. You can see all the other islands." The next day begins with a 25-mile (40 km) downhill to Punaluu State Park, not far from the island's southern tip. "This portion of the ride takes you through four or five of Hawaii's climate zones," Julie continued. "You glide from volcanic plateau to high desert with mesquite and cacti, to less arid country with larger trees on down to palms and more tropical vegetation. Punaluu is famous for its beautiful black sand beach and green sea turtles, which are almost always present. This beach is a little rocky for swimming, but at our lodging for the evening, Keauhou Beach Resort, there's one of the best snorkeling bays (Kahaluu) on the island. You can't snorkel every day of the trip, but you can get in the water five out of seven days!" In addition to fine snorkeling, Keauhou offers a rich Hawaiian culture program. "You can take crafts classes to learn to make headdresses and leis, learn the Hawaiian language, or take a guided tour of the grounds, which include one of King Kamehameha's meetinghouses and fishponds," Julie added. "It's a chance to see the island through local eyes."

The following day, you'll ride through some of the coffee plantations of Kona and on to *Pu'uhonua o Honaunau*—the City of Refuge. In older times, many infractions (like eating forbidden foods) carried the penalty of death, but there was one loophole—if you could reach Pu'uhonua o Honaunau ahead of your pursuers, you were allowed to live. "There are many *ki'i* (carved wooden images), huts, and more fishponds here," Julie said. "Sometimes there are carvers on-site building dugouts. We continue on to Waikoloa. The bike course for the annual Ironman Competition ('Swim 2.4 miles! Bike 112 miles! Run 26.2 miles! Brag for the rest of your life!') is nearby. It's hot, it's flat, and it's windy, but if you like Ironman, you salivate over the ride!" At Waikoloa, there's a chance to go whale watching and snorkeling (humpback sightings are almost a given in the winter months). From here, it's a short morning ride to the town of Hawi at the top of the island. Your circumnavigation is complete.

JULIE ROBINSON is a Washington native and came to Bicycle Adventures after more than fourteen years in sales and customer service, including work at the Starbucks Corporation and amazon.com. She enjoys running and rides regularly with her local cycling club's fixed-gear group.

If You Go

▶ **Getting There:** Riders generally depart from or near Kona, which is served by many major carriers, including Alaska Airlines (800-252-7522; www.alaskaair.com).

▶ **Best Time to Visit:** October through March is considered the dry season, though weather is always temperate—and changeable.

▶ **Guides/Outfitters:** Companies leading trips on the Big Island include Bicycle Adventures (800-443-6060; www.bicycleadventures.com) and Backroads (800-462-2848; www.backroads.com).

▶ **Level of Difficulty:** The perimeter ride entails six to seven days of riding, with an average of 45 miles (72 km) a day. It's rated moderate to difficult.

▶ **Accommodations:** Bicycle Adventures likes the following Big Island properties: in Hilo, Hilo Hawaiian Hotel (800-367-5004; www.castleresorts.com); near Volcanoes National Park, Kilauea Lodge (808-967-7366; www.kilauealodge.com); in Keauhou, Keauhou Beach Resort (866-326-6803; www.outrigger.com); and in Waikoloa, Waikoloa Beach Resort (888-236-2427; www.marriott.com).

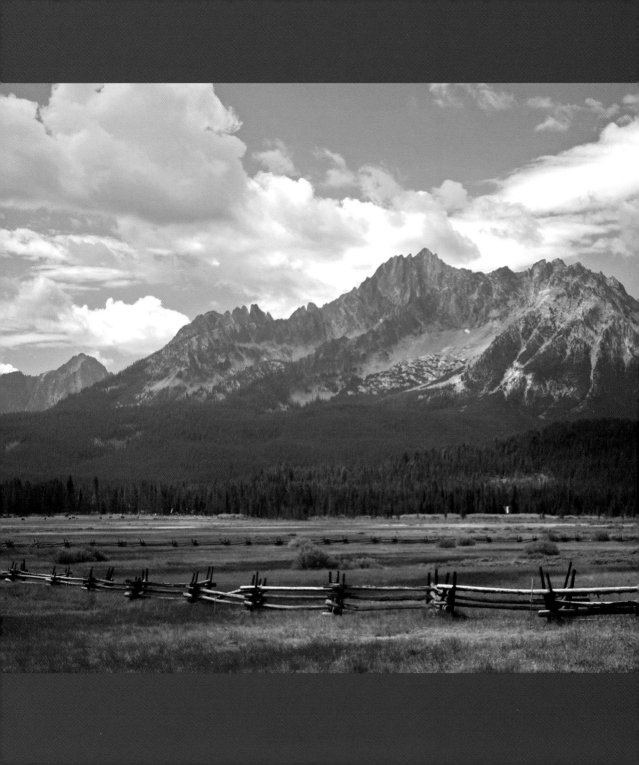

SAWTOOTH MOUNTAINS

RECOMMENDED BY **Anne St. Clair**

If you enjoy sustained climbs, majestic mountain vistas, and Old West history—along with ample natural hot springs to soothe your calves and thighs after those sustained climbs—then Idaho's Sawtooth Mountains might be just right for you! "One of the things I really enjoy about this ride is how it showcases so many different sides of Idaho," Anne St. Clair began. "You begin in Boise, Idaho's biggest city, then ride through an old gold mining town, along the edge of a wilderness area, and finally on to Sun Valley, one of the west's great outdoor recreation destinations. A big bonus is that the roads are not heavily trafficked, though they're nicely graded. If you're a true cyclist, you'll love this tour. At the end of each day you feel like you've gotten good miles in, with tremendous scenery."

Before setting out in a northeasterly direction on Highway 21 (the Ponderosa Pine Scenic Byway) toward Idaho City, take a day to poke around Boise. Boise has quietly prospered in the shadow of its larger neighbors to the west, benefiting from the tech boom and reinvesting in its compact but thriving downtown. Blessed with abundant sunshine, ample green space, a healthy river that flows through the middle of downtown to accommodate both fly anglers and kayakers, and quality skiing and mountain biking within thirty minutes of downtown, Boise has attracted many outdoor lifestyle enthusiasts. College football fans may wish to make a pilgrimage to the blue turf of Bronco Stadium, home of the Boise State squad. The city is also home to one of America's largest Basque populations; these immigrants from the Pyrenees were drawn to western Idaho to tend the vast herds of sheep that once grazed here. Their little-known culture is on display at the Basque Museum and Basque Market.

If Boise embodies the upside of a modern economic surge, the environs of Idaho City display a boomtown that's seen better days. During the peak of the Boise Basin gold rush

OPPOSITE:

The Sawtooth
Mountains near
Stanley, Idaho,
and Redfish Lake.

in the early 1860s, Idaho City boasted more than 250 businesses, from opera houses to bowling alleys—and of course, saloons. By 1865, Idaho City had surpassed Portland as the Pacific Northwest's largest city. However, by 1870 the gold deposits had dwindled, and most of Idaho City's population had moved on. "It's a gem of an authentic small Idaho mountain town, with rich gold rush history!" Anne continued. "It's not overly commercialized, and it still holds its small-town charm. We usually roll in, get some huckleberry ice cream or homemade pie, and then hike up to the Pioneer Cemetery. It's interesting to see how different immigrant populations are grouped together; it reflects the settlement patterns of the area."

The next day brings the first of the route's sustained climbs—2,500 feet over 13 miles (21 km)—up to Banner Ridge. "The grades are steep, but doable," Anne described. "You spin and spin, you get in your groove, work hard and sweat, and then you're at the top, and you're surrounded by the Boise National Forest." Descending from Banner Ridge, you'll reach Kirkham Hot Springs, along the Payette River. "Kirkham has a number of different pools," Anne continued. "The farther down, the cooler the pools are. One is shaped like a large, deep hot tub. In some spots, the water pours down like a shower—it gives you a great shoulder massage. The river is cold; if levels are not too high, it can be very invigorating to jump in from rocks upstream and float down to the springs. (Exercise good judgment!) It's easy to spend most of the afternoon relaxing around the springs. Our next stop is at either Warm Springs or Bonneville, where even more hot springs await." (Idaho, incidentally, can claim some 130 "soakable" hot springs—that is, springs that are not too hot for humans. Most of the hot springs in Idaho—as well as the geothermal activity in Yellowstone—are believed to have resulted from energy that was generated from a meteor that crashed into present-day southeast Oregon some seventeen million years ago.)

With Banner Ridge under your belt, you'll tackle another big climb on day three, the 30-mile (48-km) ascent to Banner Summit, which rests at more than 7,000 feet. Today you'll get your first glimpse of the Sawtooths, part of the northern Rockies, with forty peaks above 10,000 feet. You'll want to include a few stops along the way to snap photos, and be sure to keep your camera handy as you descend into Stanley, staging ground for white-water, backpacking, and other adventures in the Sawtooth National Recreation Area, which sets aside more than 750,000 acres for outdoor play. After an ice cream or bakery treat, it's a few more miles to Redfish Lake, a 5-mile-long glacial lake nestled in the

DESTINATION 18

Sawtooths. The lake takes its name from the sockeye salmon that used to return some 900 miles from the Pacific to spawn here in considerable numbers. Dams on the Columbia and Snake River systems nearly drove Redfish Lake sockeye to extinction; some might recall "Lonesome Larry," the single salmon that returned to the lake in 1991. Larry's story galvanized government efforts to resuscitate the run, and thanks to the Redfish Lake Sockeye Captive Broodstock Program, more than 1,200 fish returned to the lake in 2010. Redfish Lake is a great layover spot. There's an old family resort on the water that rents canoes and kayaks and serves cold beer on a shaded deck. There's also the option of an exhilarating rafting trip on the nearby Salmon River or a hike around the lake. Or you can hop back on your bike and go hot spring hunting toward the town of Clayton along the Salmon. Of course, after the previous day's 4,000-plus feet of climbing, reclining in an Adirondack chair with a good book and mountain view might be about right. "Every time I get to Redfish Lake, I'm in awe of Mount Heyburn, which rises 10,299 feet up behind it," Anne added.

Sun Valley is the next stop on your route. To get there you'll climb through the Idaho backcountry to the Galena Summit (8,795 feet). "As you're nearing the pinnacle of the climb, you can look down and see the headwaters of the East Fork of the Salmon River," Anne said. "It always gives me pause—to think of the long route the river takes, how it connects to the larger drainage and eventually makes it to the sea. From Galena, we have a last wilderness hurrah—a 30-mile (48-km) descent back to civilization. Down in Ketchum, you have all the amenities again—including bike shops if serious repairs are needed." (Ernest Hemingway, among other celebrities, was invited to the Ketchum area as part of the Sun Valley Company's efforts to promote the region as a summer/fall getaway in the mid-1930s. He would take his life here in 1961.) There's a nice system of bike paths to ease you back into the idea of traffic. After an evening of wandering the downtown, you can follow the bike paths through Hailey and Bellevue, before dropping down to Highway 20. The ride ends at the Silver Creek Preserve, which protects one of the West's great trout streams—an endeavor initiated by Ernest's son, Jack.

ANNE ST. CLAIR is a mountain bike and road cycling tour guide for Escape Adventures. Anne first discovered her love for two-wheeled transport after her graduation from the University of Notre Dame when she rode across the United States from New Haven, Connecticut, to Seattle, Washington, to raise money and awareness for Habitat for

Humanity. The thrill of exploration combined with the physical and mental challenge amid the simplicity of life on the open road was something she decided to make more than a hobby when she joined the team at Escape Adventures. As a full-time multiday guide, Anne travels the northern and southwestern United States leading groups on four- to seven-day mountain biking and road cycling tours. When she is not guiding, Anne can be found at local downhill mountain bike races or scheming up endurance rides and bike tours of her own from Ometepe, Nicaragua, and Copper Canyon, Mexico, to her backyard in Moab, Utah. In the off-season, Anne explores the Colorado Rockies on skis from her base camp in Breckenridge.

If You Go

► **Getting There:** The trip described here begins and ends in the Idaho state capital in Boise, which is served by many carriers.

► **Best Time to Visit:** The passes will generally be clear from June through September.

► **Guides/Outfitters:** There are several tour companies that lead rides through the Sawtooths, including Escape Adventures (800-596-2953; www.escapeadventures.com).

► **Level of Difficulty:** This tour involves six days of riding, with an average 35 miles (56 km) a day. It's rated moderate.

► **Accommodations:** Some riders will choose to camp on this excursion. If you prefer a softer bed, some lodging options include: Idaho City Hotel (208-392-4499; http://idahocitylodge.com) in Idaho City, Sourdough Lodge (208-259-3326; www.sourdough lodge.com) in Lowman, Red Fish Lake Lodge (208-774-3536; www.redfishlake.com) near Stanley, and Sun Valley Inn (800-786-8259; www.sunvalley.com).

BALI

RECOMMENDED BY **Emile Leushuis**

Bali is a seductive, tropical land of steep volcanic mountains, pristine beaches of white and black sand, and warm Indonesian hospitality. Until recently, honeymooners and scuba divers have helped sustain a significant tourism trade that subsidizes the island's core agricultural economy based on the cultivation of rice. Now bicycle travelers are beginning to appear on the island, perhaps signaling a new tourism trend.

"I've run Djoser's tours around Bali and the neighboring island of Lombok for twenty years," Emile Leushuis explained, "and it's a fascinating place. There are incredible beaches, active volcanoes, and a vibrant agrarian lifestyle. Bali is the only Hindu culture in Southeast Asia, which sets it apart from the rest of Indonesia, which is predominantly Islamic. Lombok has both Hindu and Islamic communities. The whole package makes this area of Indonesia attractive.

"After many years of leading cultural tours for Djoser, we developed bike tours on Bali and Lombok. It's been surprising to me how different the experience is. We get to remote places you just don't reach in a car or bus—little villages, rice fields, isolated beaches. Residents in some of these off-the-beaten-path places don't see many foreigners, let alone strangers on bicycles. When twenty westerners on bikes show up, the locals get very excited. It's not an interaction you'd have on a coach tour. I'm always amazed at how open the Indonesians are toward outsiders. Asia is a warm blanket in general, but Indonesia is even more welcoming. People might be a little shy in out-of-the-way places, but once the ice is broken, they're very warm and inviting."

Emile pointed out that most of the biking days on the Bali and Lombok tour are not that long—a half-day or so. "Biking on Bali and Lombok is really about experiencing the nature and culture of the islands," he noted. "During the bike trips, we rumble through

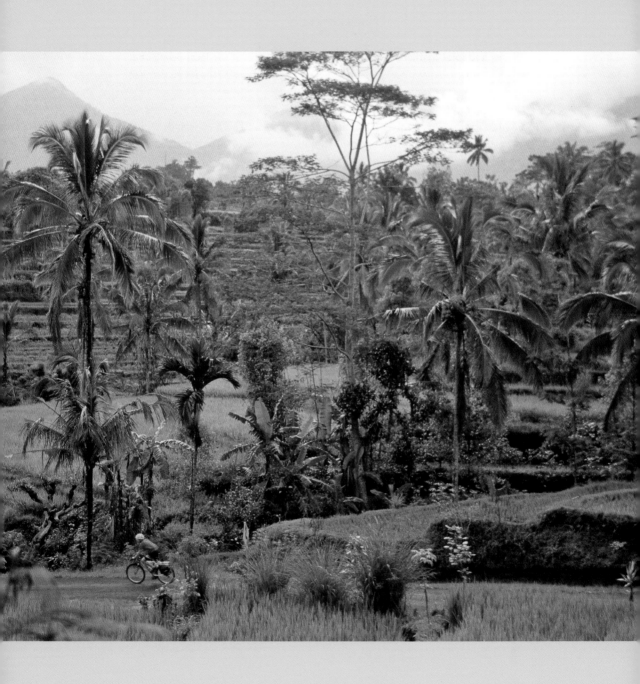

small villages and local markets and experience the way of life of the local people, but besides that, we always leave time to do hikes, visit the beach, snorkel the reefs, and visit temples and other cultural sites."

Bali and Lombok are two of Indonesia's thirty-three provinces, lying just to the east of Java, and a few degrees south of the equator. The volcanic nature of both islands makes their soil exceptionally fertile; several volcanic mountains on both islands rise dramatically from sea level to higher than 10,000 feet. Bali and Lombok were colonized by the Dutch in the second half of the nineteenth century, the Dutch East India Company having been established in the region in the early 1600s to facilitate trade. After a brief occupation by the Japanese during World War II, Bali and Lombok became part of Indonesia after it declared its independence from the Dutch in 1945. The Dutch assented to the change in 1949.

Visitors generally fly into the international airport in Denpasar, Bali. From there, Emile likes to shuttle them to Ubud in the center of the island, which is recognized as Bali's cultural capital, thanks to a concentration of artists and the presence of several key Hindu temples. Here, one has a chance to observe the vibrant Balinese brand of Hinduism, which differs from the religion practiced in other parts of the world, combining elements of animism, Buddhism, ancestor worship, and traditional Hinduism. While visiting Ubud, you may wish to hike through one of the area's exquisitely terraced rice fields or take a walk through the Monkey Forest. The Monkey Forest is considered a sacred site, for its ravines and thick copses (which are believed to harbor human and animal spirits) as well as for several temples. As the name implies, it is also home to more than three hundred long-tailed macaque monkeys, which wander the woods in troops.

Your cycling begins in earnest as you head toward the mountains in northwestern Bali and then move across the north and east coasts. Starting on the slopes of Mount Batukaru, you'll weave up and down along a tropical rain forest habitat that's dotted with cocoa, coffee, and clove plantations; you'll smell the clove before you spot the plantation! You'll pass the Pura Batukaru temple, another important Hindu site, and visit the rice fields at Jatiluwih, which unfold in green undulations toward the sea. Given the many rice fields in Bali, it's no surprise that rice is a staple. "Meals typically feature some vegetables, tofu, and some duck, fish, or chicken," Emile added. "But it's mostly rice. As a saying goes, 'if there isn't any rice in it, it isn't a meal.'"

OPPOSITE:
In Bali, you're
never far from
rice paddies.

After an overnight stay in the mountain village of Munduk, you'll ride downhill toward the beaches of the north coast. "Riding through the villages, you'll often come upon residents participating in Hindu ceremonies of one sort or another," Emile continued. "On one occasion, we were riding down to the coast from Munduk, and there was a very large celebration going on in a private home with a number of people. Our biking group was all invited inside, even though we were in our bike clothing and everyone else was in ceremonial gear. We didn't look the way we should have for such a formal event, but everyone was incredibly open and friendly."

In keeping with the notion of a multifaceted Balinese exploration, Emile likes to spend a few days in the seaside resort of Lovina. "Some visitors will take a boat out to spot bottlenose dolphins," Emile said. "There's also a coral reef just offshore that provides first-rate snorkeling and diving." Indeed, the waters off Bali are celebrated for their marine life; it's not uncommon for divers to encounter bumphead parrotfish, manta rays, sea snakes, and hammerhead shark. Returning to the saddle, you'll continue along the coast to the east, passing more black and white sand beaches as well as the traditional production of salt from seawater. Gunung Agung, the highest point on Bali at 10,308 feet, looms in the distance; the volcano last erupted in 1963, destroying many surrounding villages. After spending the night in the seaside village of Amed, riders encounter the hilliest terrain of the tour while traversing the island in a southeasterly direction toward the coastal town of Padangbai: a beautiful ride that sums up all the exquisiteness of Bali. From here, you can ferry to the adjoining island of Lombok for a few more days of touring. "Lombok is quite different from Bali," Emile added. "It's a poorer island overall, partly Hindu and partly Islamic. People dress differently and have different customs, but it is just as vibrant and authentic and welcoming to visitors."

EMILE LEUSHUIS is a Dutch national who has acted as the Indonesia representative for Djoser Inc. since 1991, leading international groups for Dutch and North American travelers. With great enthusiasm, in addition to the Djoser biking tours, he has guided hundreds of Djoser's cultural tours around the many islands of the archipelago. Bali and Lombok are longtime favorites, although nowadays, he resides in Yogyakarta on the island of Java. He has written for magazines and published several books about his many experiences in Indonesia.

If You Go

▶ **Getting There:** Most visitors to Bali fly into the international airport at Denpasar, which is reachable via Los Angeles on a number of carriers, including China Airlines (800-227-5118; www.china-airlines.com) and Cathay Pacific (800-233-2742; www.cathaypacific.com).

▶ **Best Time to Visit:** Bali is almost sure to be dry between April and October; December and January tend to be the wettest months.

▶ **Guides/Outfitters:** Djoser USA (877-356-7376; www.djoserusa.com) is among the first outfitters to lead bike-oriented tours of Bali.

▶ **Level of Difficulty:** The Bali section of this trip entails five days of riding over nine days, with rides between 15 and 24 miles (24 and 39 km). It's rated moderate.

▶ **Accommodations:** The Bali Tourism Board (www.balitourismboard.org) lists lodging options around the island. Lombok Tourism (www.lombok-tourism.com) highlights options on that island.

19

DESTINATION

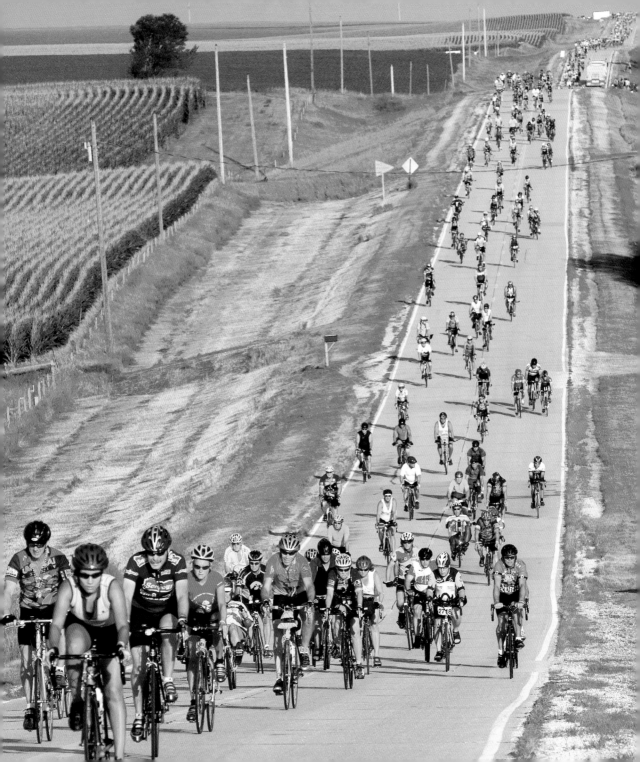

RAGBRAI®

RECOMMENDED BY **T.J. Juskiewicz**

RAGBRAI: To the uninitiated, it sounds like a computer virus or a covert intelligence operation. To Iowans in even the smallest hamlets—and to thousands of cyclists around the world—it means the Register's Annual Great Bicycle Ride Across Iowa, a seven-day bicycle journey across the Hawkeye State that's been going strong since 1973.

"There's a simple formula that makes RAGBRAI special," T.J. Juskiewicz began. "It's the people who open their towns and their hearts to visitors. We don't necessarily have the greatest scenery—there are lots of corn and soybean fields—but the welcome that people receive blows them away, from the seventy-five-year-old lady baking pies to the kids squirting water guns at overheated riders. It's the state's event—no matter where the ride goes, the hospitality is incredible. There are some 900 towns in the state of Iowa; for 890 of those towns, RAGBRAI is the largest event they'll ever host. At least ten thousand people roll into town. Some years it's closer to twenty-five thousand bicyclists. There are many rides that have emulated RAGBRAI. But I don't think they can but emulate the hospitality."

RAGBRAI was born in 1973 when columnist Don Kaul and copyeditor John Karras from the *Des Moines Register* decided to ride across the state and write a series of columns describing the trip. They invited readers to join them, and 115 people rode the entire distance. "One of the most interesting people the ride attracted was Clarence Pickard, an eighty-three-year-old man from Indianola, Iowa," T.J. continued. "Clarence had a woman's touring Schwinn—a very heavy bike—and rode all the way from Sioux City to Davenport, clad in a long-sleeved shirt, woolen long underwear, and a pith helmet. Clarence's success showed the public that with a little determination, anyone could do the ride. Cycling was not as popular at this time—people were more into running. But each year the event grew, and by the tenth year, we had ten thousand riders."

OPPOSITE: Some years, as many as twenty-five thousand riders partake of Iowa hospitality during RABGRAI.

RAGBRAI unfolds over seven days, and generally totals 472 miles (760 km). The route taken varies each year, with the goal of bringing the ride's circus atmosphere to every town that desires a visit—which covers most of them. One constant is that the ride moves from west (somewhere along the Missouri River) to east (somewhere along the Mississippi) so riders can take advantage of prevailing winds. Outsiders who have the perception of Iowa as pancake flat are generally surprised at the heartland's pleasantly rolling topography. "We have many rivers in Iowa, and the watersheds create some spectacular bluffs, especially along the Mississippi," T.J. said. "On the western side of the state, you have the Loess Hills—not exactly the Rockies, but they create a nice challenge for riders. Thanks to the breadth of the ride and the changing itineraries, cyclists have the chance to see every nook and cranny of the state. We've ridden by the fields where the movie *Field of Dreams* was filmed, and riders have stopped to hit a few baseballs. We've been over the bridges of Madison County. But the best moments are when you pull into a tiny town, and residents begin breaking out the corn and watermelons. It's like a Fourth of July celebration every day of the ride, a slice of Americana."

As the population of some hosting towns is dwarfed by the entourage of riders that descends upon them, nearly all participants camp out. T.J. described a typical day. "You'll likely wake up in a tent, maybe on a farm, maybe in someone's yard. After packing your duffel bag, tent, and sleeping bag, you begin down the road. In 5 miles (8 km) or so, there will be a small church serving waffles or pancakes. Ten miles farther along, there's a band playing in the town square. You might stop to dance or have a piece of pie. The next town might have a beer garden set up, and a little museum that's worth a stop. The next town, a spread of pork chops and corn. Eventually you get to the town where you'll be staying. If you're staying in someone's yard, you might join your host family for a glass of lemonade or a beer on the porch. Dinner will be in a downtown church or banquet hall that's serving meat loaf or beef and noodles—or more pork tenderloins, chops, and corn—all cooked by volunteers. There will be more music that night, sometimes a local band, sometimes a national act like Barenaked Ladies. The next morning, you wake up and do it all again.

"If you took a poll of the favorite food items on the trip, the pies would probably come out near the top. Strawberry rhubarb, cherry, apple, boysenberry, bumbleberry, all with homemade crust. Outside a VFW hall, you might have a football field's length of pies. If you're riding almost 500 miles (800 km) over a week, you're using some calories. Still, if you're not gaining a little weight by the end of the trip, you're not doing it right!"

RAGBRAI has entertained a few Tour de France champions, and no shortage of people who can barely ride. They all get the red carpet treatment from their Iowa hosts. "We've had some folks from out of state who come back every year," T.J. reflected. "They can't put their finger on why they're spending their vacation in Iowa instead of Hawaii, but they're here. I think it's because RAGBRAI provides a chance to revert to a simpler life, a chance to visit with and get to know people who share a love of biking. You're not worrying about the stock market or Facebook or e-mail. Your biggest concern is whether you'll get to the next town before the last piece of pie is sold.

"There's a euphoria that's hard to explain when you pull into a town with fifty tractors lined up, kids waving flags and cheering. It's a very emotional experience."

T.J. JUSKIEWICZ is the director of RAGBRAI, Register's Annual Great Bicycle Ride Across Iowa®. He has also served as director of Florida's cross-state ride, Bike Florida, and has been involved with the event since its inaugural ride in 1992. T.J. helped coordinate Bike South 2000, a 2,000-mile (3,219 km), thirty-day bicycle tour of six southern states. Prior to his work in the cycling industry, he served as director of Florida's Sunshine State Games, the state's Olympic-style multisport festival. He also worked at the Olympic Games in Atlanta and in the University of Florida athletic department.

If You Go

▶ **Getting There:** RAGBRAI always begins in western Iowa and ends on the eastern edge of the state. There are charter services that can get you from Des Moines, Chicago, or St. Louis to the beginning point of the ride and then transfer you back from the ending point. Visit the RAGBRAI website (http://ragbrai.com) for details.

▶ **Best Time to Visit:** RAGBRAI is held the last week of July each year. Visit the RAGBRAI website (http://ragbrai.com) for details and registration information.

▶ **Level of Difficulty:** RAGBRAI covers 472 miles (760 km) over seven days. It's rated moderate for people who cycle regularly.

▶ **Accommodations:** Most participants camp out during RAGBRAI. Travel Iowa (www.traveliowa.com) lists lodging options around the state.

20 DESTINATION

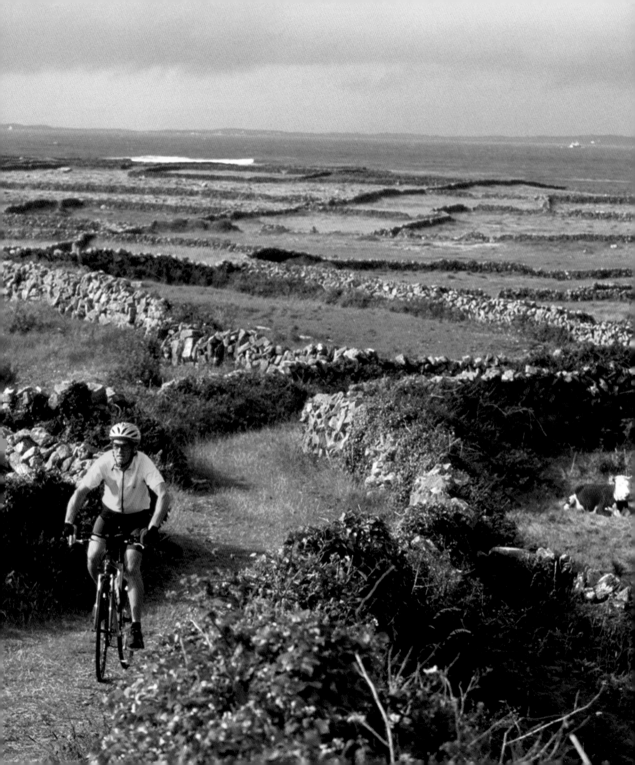

CONNEMARA

RECOMMENDED BY **Catherine Dowling**

"There is something magical about the west of Ireland," Catherine Dowling enthused. "It's a fairly desolate landscape. Some might call it bleak, but it's bleak in a romantic way. Those wide-open melancholic spaces really do uplift the soul. The topography is hilly, and it looks different each time I ride, depending on the light and the mist. The drama of the scenery is only part of the appeal. We pass through many small towns, and the people there are eager to chat. With the exception of Galway, it's a very rural region, and people are not in a rush. There's a genuine kindness amongst them. I swear their hearts beat at a much slower rate, and I always get lots of belly laughter. Cyclists here have to be ready for a good dollop of rain and wind," Catherine added. "But I like to think that the warmth of the citizenry balances that out."

Your ride will begin in County Clare and take you through the Burren ("rocky coast" in Gaelic), a region of limestone karst that's been likened to a moonscape. Oliver Cromwell famously described the Burren as a place where "there's not a tree whereon to hang a man; no water in which to drown him; no soil in which to bury him." (Cromwell, of course, hoped to hang and drown the Irish, whom he was attempting to conquer and colonize.) A closer look, however, may reveal wildflowers growing in the sheltered crevices of limestone—saxifrages, orchids, and rockroses, to name a few; this is one of the few places in the world where arctic, Mediterranean, and alpine plants thrive side by side. A careful eye might also notice ancient dolmens (rock tombs). "One dolmen I like to visit is called Poulnabrone, or 'hole of sorrows,'" Catherine continued. "Prehistoric peoples buried their dead in these simple structures of upright stones. Many were drawn to the area; some believe it was considered a place of healing or had some spiritual significance. We can only imagine that it was a harsh existence." Near the northern edge of the Burren,

OPPOSITE:
The history of
western Ireland
is told in part
by its ancient
stone walls.

the road veers close to the sea. By the time you reach Black Head—the tip of the peninsula—the Atlantic is on your left and the Burren Peaks, a series of small mountains, are to your right in a classic Irish cycling vista.

After a morning ride past medieval churches and the Corcomroe Abbey, a Cistercian monastery dating to the early thirteenth century, you'll continue to the lively university city of Galway. You may wish to take a meal in the Quays Bar, a traditional Guinness and oyster pub (Galway is celebrated for its oysters, thanks in part to the long-running Galway International Oyster Festival). You'll board a ferry the next morning bound for Inishmore, the largest of the Aran Islands at the western edge of Galway Bay. (Some may know the Arans for their namesake cable-knit sweaters.) "Inishmore is the most populated of the islands—perhaps eight hundred people," Catherine said. "Tourism is important to the folk here in the summer, but the rest of the year they make their living from fishing and farming. As you ride around the island, you'll notice hundreds of miles of stone walls. Some were built when the Romans were invading; more were built in the nineteenth century to mark property boundaries—especially after the English came. It was a way for the Irish to say, 'This is my territory.' One must-see spot on Inishmore is Dun Aengus, a Druid site that dates back more than three thousand years. No matter what your belief system, it's impossible not to be moved. The site is very grand, and the very impressive cliffs with the crashing and thundering waves below can be very humbling. A remarkable network of defensive stones known as a cheval-de-frise surrounds the whole structure. It's eerie, but eerie in a beautiful way. The ground there holds a lot of power."

Returning to the mainland at Rossaveal, you'll cycle north to Connemara. The country here is framed by the Twelve Bens mountain range and Roundstone Bog, a peat bog. "The Twelve Bens are not very high—the tallest of the lot (Benbaun) is only 2,392 feet," Catherine continued, "but they're enchanting. At times in the warmer months the heather and gorse on the hills are in flower, and they glow gold and fuchsia. Visitors are often curious about the peat bogs and the role they play in Irish life. There are two types of bogs—blanket bogs in the coastal areas (like Roundstone) and raised bogs in the interior. They're both made up of dying vegetation that's rotted and sunk into the waterlogged soil. When this vegetative matter condenses, it becomes peat. Peat has been used for fuel since the seventeenth century (and still is used in rural areas today); it's called turf when it's cut. It's estimated that 15 percent of Ireland's bogs have been destroyed by cutting, though efforts are being made to limit the peat harvest to preserve these unique ecosystems."

After a day of riding the "wild west" of Connemara, you'll likely be seeking a bit of warmth and nourishment. What better place to find such succor than a true Irish pub. "Most of the pubs in Connemara are of the 'old-school' type," Catherine described, "where locals come in to socialize and tell stories. These quirky characters are always up for a conversation. The drink of choice is Guinness stout or whiskey (Irish, of course). As for pub food, seafood chowder is quite common given Connemara's place on the Atlantic. Bacon and cabbage is another favorite dish. Visitors always comment about how good the food is. Irish food has had a poor reputation, but culinary tastes and habits are vastly improved in the past twenty years."

CATHERINE DOWLING lives in Dublin, and has been leading tours with VBT since 2006.

If You Go

▶ **Getting There:** Most guests will fly into Shannon.

▶ **Best Time to Visit:** It's often moist around Connemara, but May through September sees slightly warmer weather and a better chance for sun.

▶ **Guides/Outfitters:** Several companies lead tours along Ireland's west coast, including VBT (800-245-3868; www.vbt.com).

▶ **Level of Difficulty:** This ride is rated easy to moderate, with an average of 28 miles (45 km) a day over five days of riding.

▶ **Accommodations:** VBT likes the following properties: in Ennis, Old Ground Hotel (+35 3 65 682 8127; www.flynnhotels.com); in Lisdoonvarna, Sheedy's Country House Hotel and Restaurant (+353 65 707 4026; www.sheedys.com); in Galway, Park House Hotel (+353 91 564924; www.parkhousehotel.ie); in Inishmore, Kilmurvey Guesthouse (+353 0 99 61218; www.kilmurveyhouse.com); in Connemara, Lough Inagh Lodge (+353 095 34706; www.loughinaghlodgehotel.ie).

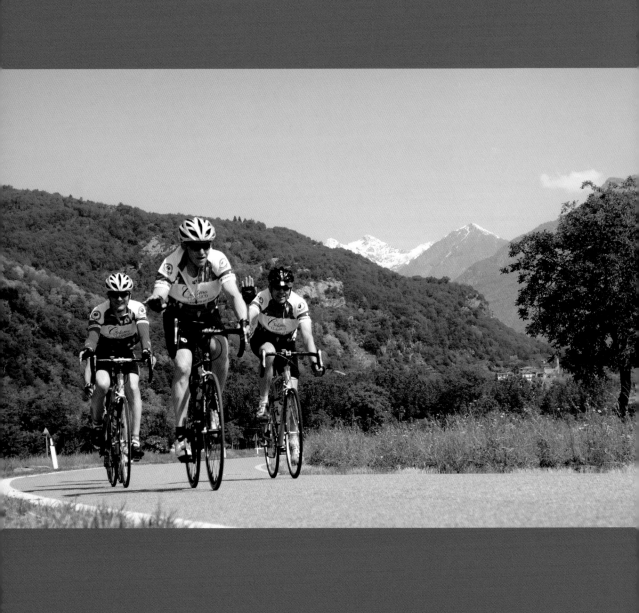

PIEDMONT

RECOMMENDED BY **Cristiano Bonino**

"There are twenty regions in Italy, and each has a different food, wine, history, and culture," Cristiano Bonino began. "Each region is special, but I have a great affinity for Piedmont as my home turf. I believe that anyone who enjoys fine food and wine will appreciate what we have to offer. The slow food movement began here (in the town of Bra) in the late 1980s, and people are still committed to the tradition of family recipes handed down from mother to daughter, small-scale food production, and the importance of a simple meal with friends. Wine lovers might know the Piedmont for the 'three Bs'—Barolo, Barbera, and Barbaresco. Yet there are a number of other native grapes that people may not know, and during a week's visit, you might sample fifteen to twenty different varietals you won't likely find anywhere else. From a cycling perspective, the area where I like to ride has spectacular views of vineyards at almost every turn. Even in May before the grapes have appeared, the tidy rows of vines are very nice. There's rolling terrain for the most part, with just enough 1-mile climbs so you feel you've earned a hearty lunch. Piedmont doesn't see as many tourists as some parts of Italy. The roads are generally quiet, and we move from sleepy village to sleepy village without competing with buses full of visitors when we visit a winery. You can have a very personal experience with the winemakers."

One of Cristiano's favorite Piedmont rides focuses on the southeastern segment of the region, with stops in Gavi, Acqui Terme, Alba, and Moncalvo. He described the wines that are sampled on the route.

"The Barbera is one of our best-known grapes, the equivalent of the Chianti grape in Tuscany," Cristiano explained. "It used to be the grape of daily wine for farmers, a quaffing wine. In the last ten or twenty years, it's become more stylish. The Barolo and Barbaresco are both made from the Nebbiolo grape and are in general aged longer.

OPPOSITE:
The Piedmont, in
the shadow of the
Alps, serves up
quiet roads and
culinary delights.

107

There's not much use of small oak barrels here, as winemakers try to maintain the flavors of the grape and soil. There's also not so much blending. Wines are usually made with one type of grape. Piedmont is known for its dessert wines as well. Moscato goes wonderfully with cookies and custard-based sweets. Barolo Chinato, which is made using Barolo wine mixed with herbs and quinine, is wonderful with chocolate. There are several wines that visitors might not be as well acquainted with. The Grignolino is very commonly served in Piedmont; it's a cherry red wine that pairs well with fish. While Piedmont is not celebrated for whites, there are several fine grapes grown here—the Cortese (used in the Gavi) and the Arneis grape. The remnants of the various crushes—just skins and pips— are recycled by a number of producers to make grappa."

Near the vineyards of Barolo and Monforte, there's another treasure that awaits—*tartufo bianco*, the white truffle. Fall is the season when truffles appear. Look for them in late September. The supply reaches its peak in late October and November. Cyclists who visit Piedmont at this time of year can take part in the fungi-fueled fervor that climaxes with *Fiera International del Tartufo Bianco*, the International Truffle Fair. "This is one of the few places in the world where white truffles grow, and they are like magic," Cristiano enthused. "It's impossible for humans to spot them; you need a specially trained dog. Trainers can tell when the dogs are puppies if they have what it takes to be a champ. It's funny that something that's resting underground in rotting leaves has come to be so valued—costing up to a thousand dollars a pound. Chemical tests have shown that white truffles contain pheromones, though scientific research hasn't yet proved any real aphrodisiac effect! White truffles have an intense garlic-like flavor. In Piedmont, they are used primarily in four dishes: shaved on a plate with flat egg noodles dressed with melted butter; shaved on a sunny-side-up egg; shaved on raw Fassone beef that's been drizzled with olive oil; and shaved over local Robiola di Roccaverano cheese."

When asked about more of the Piedmont's most renowned dishes, Cristiano did not hesitate. "We have a ravioli or dumpling called *agnolotti*, filled with ground beef. It's traditionally served with *sugo d'arrosto*, the juice from slowly braised beef. Some will eat *agnolotti* the ancient way, dressed with a splash of wine. We're also well-known for our antipasti or appetizers. One is *vitello tonnato*, thinly sliced veal dressed with a sauce of mayonnaise flavored with tuna. Another is raw ground Fassone beef, dressed with a drop of olive oil and a couple drops of lemon, a pinch of salt and pepper. Perhaps our most famous dish is *bagna cauda*, a 'hot sauce' made with lots of garlic and carefully cleaned anchovies. These ingredients are slowly cooked in an earthenware container. Everything melts down to a paste, then it's combined with olive oil. The *bagna cauda* is used as a dipping sauce with vegetables. It's pretty intense—you're unapproachable for a few days!

"For me, some of the most special moments on a trip to Piedmont are those when we can really interact with the local people. One of my colleagues, Enrico, has a friend who owns a small winery near Nizza Monferrato. The family opens its doors to our group, and we have lunch in their living room. The mamma serves locally made salami, a savory vegetable tart or bell peppers dressed with an anchovy sauce, and tastings of the different wines the family makes. It's a two-hour lunch, something that many American guests aren't used to. But I think everyone agrees that it's magical."

CRISTIANO BONINO is a trip specialist and tour consultant for Ciclismo Classico. A native of Piedmont, Italy, he is a former marathon runner, avid cyclist, a locavore foodie who is passionate about cooking, and an optimist to the core. Cristiano has biked all over Italy and parts of France, Slovenia, Croatia, and the United States, and currently leads rides on ten different itineraries in Italy and France, including Piedmont, Sardinia and Corsica, Puglia, Tuscany and Umbria, Friuli and Slovenia, Dordogne, and Provence.

If You Go

▶ **Getting There:** Most visitors to Piedmont fly into Milan.

▶ **Best Time to Visit:** May through October, though August may be hot for some travelers.

▶ **Guides/Outfitters:** A number of tour companies lead trips through the Piedmont, including Ciclismo Classico (800-866-7314; www.ciclismoclassico.com).

▶ **Level of Difficulty:** The trip above covers 238 miles (383 km) over seven days. It's rated moderate.

▶ **Accommodations:** Ciclismo Classico likes the following properties: in Monterotondo di Gavi, L'Ostelliere Albergo (+39 0143 607801; www.ostelliere.it); in Acqui Terme, The Grand Hotel Nuove Terme (+39 0144 58555; www.grandhotelacquiterme.it); in Alba, Palazzo Finati (+39 0173 366324; www.palazzofinati.it); in Penango, Relais il Borgo da Beppe (+39 0141 921 272; www.ilborgodicioccaro.com).

DESTINATION 22

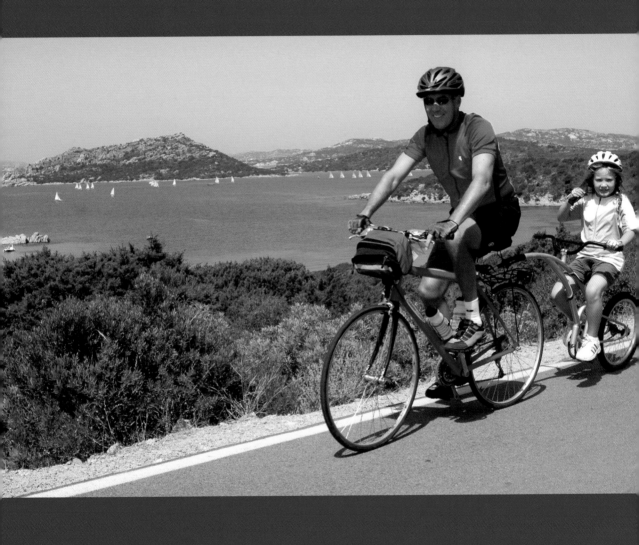

SARDINIA

RECOMMENDED BY **Lauren Hefferon**

"I studied archaeology and anthropology in college, and I love places with great architecture and culture," Lauren Hefferon began. "I came to Italy to continue my education. When I was living in Italy, I'd ask the people I'd meet, 'Where are the great places to ride?' After I heard about a place, I'd go to a bookstore and look at maps and guidebooks to figure it out. I was committed to riding all the great places I was learning about. When someone mentioned Sardinia, it piqued my interest. The photographs convinced me to go. Sardinia is to Italians as Hawaii is to Americans—an island Shangri-la. I love islands, the idea that you can cycle around or across and get a sense of completion. When I visited in 1992, I was blown away by how gorgeous it was. The roads were fabulous, and the contrast between the coast and the interior was tremendous. At that time, Americans knew little of Sardinia. I felt like people would embrace it, both for fitness riding and for the chance to combine swimming and biking and the opportunity to immerse yourself in an authentic, exotic culture."

Sardinia is the second-largest island in the Mediterranean Sea (160 miles long and 68 miles wide), located west of the Italian mainland, north of Tunisia and the African continent, and just south of the French island of Corsica. Throughout history, Sardinia has had a variety of courtiers and conquerors, including (but not limited to) the Phoenicians, Carthaginians, Romans, Byzantines, and finally, the Italians. The island has been part of Italy since the early 1700s, and though Italian is widely spoken and many aspects of Italian culture have been adopted, Sardinian (an early Romance language dating back two thousand years) is still commonly heard. Sardinia boasts 1,200 miles of coastline along the Tyrrhenian and Mediterranean Seas, with myriad white sand beaches and turquoise water that cries out to swimmers. Costa Smeralda (or the "Emerald Coast") on Sardinia's

OPPOSITE:
Sardinia offers
a special blend
of coastal vistas
and mountain
communities
little impacted
by modernity.

northeastern shore appeals to European jet-setters, royals, and other glitterati; it's a major stop on the Rolex Cup sailing circuit. Inland, you'll find a much different side of Sardinia—canyons dotted with ancient mountain villages, forests of chestnut and cork trees, and shepherds herding their flocks much as they have for thousands of years.

"The Sardinians have an ancient form of singing," Lauren added. "It's a very deep and living culture. All the food is sourced locally. There's a flat bread that you find around the island that's baked to be crispy, seasoned with salt and garlic. On the coast, you see mostly fish and other seafood. In the interior, there's more lamb and fresh produce; roasted pig is a specialty."

Each day's ride on Sardinia holds special surprises. Cycling north and west from Alghero to Capo Caccia, you can visit Grotta di Nettuno (Neptune's Grotto) if you are willing to descend the 656 steps down to the sea caves. Upon arrival you're treated to an arresting array of stalactites and stalagmites. "I also love the ride south from Alghero to Bosa," Lauren continued. "It's a very twisting, winding road along the amazingly blue Mediterranean, with mountains to the left. There's a more direct route for cars if they're in a hurry. The scenery reminds me of Route 1 in southern California—except for the lack of cars. There are brilliant rock formations that change at every curve. The coastline around Bosa is home to great bird life; you might come upon a reed warbler or a griffon vulture."

One of Lauren's favorite rides climbs from near the center of Sardinia, over Genna Silana pass, and then heads back down to the sea on the island's east coast. "We start from the village of Oleina, which is known for a style of Grenache wine, Cannonau di Sardegna," Lauren explained. "There's a four-star hotel there, Hotel Su Gologone, that's been run by the same family for generations. It's right at the foot of Supramonte Mountain. (The nearby village of Mamoiada is known for its ritual of the Mamuthones, which celebrates the passing of winter to spring and dates back to pre-Christian times. Participants don a black sheepskin, nearly seventy pounds of bronze cowbells, and, most famously, a dark wooden mask that's both eerie and iconic before parading through the streets.) The climb is very gradual, along a zigzagging road carved into the ridge of the mountains. To the right, you're looking out at the highlands of Supramonte. Below there's a plunging river gorge. You gain 3,280 feet, but as it's over 12 miles (19 km), you barely notice. The descent to the coast is perhaps even more dramatic, though not too steep. You come down to sea level over the course of 20 miles (32 km). You put out some energy over the day, but not too much.

"I recall my first visit to Sardinia," Lauren added. "I met a local guy, and he took me to his home. His mother was so excited to have a visitor from America in her house, she insisted that I try on her wedding gown. It was very traditional garb, with multiple layers of ornate colors and gold work. I even put on makeup, which is not typical for me. Then we had a great feast of roasted suckling pig, ravioli with fresh ricotta, *pane carasau* (Sardinian flat bread), fresh gnocchi, homemade Mirto (a Sardinian after-dinner drink), and so much more. On another occasion when I was leading a tour, we did an invigorating ride that ended on the beach. It was so great to get a good workout and then play in the waves of that beautiful water. Afterward, we took the support van to a town where there was a festival in progress. People were promenading in their ceremonial clothing, and we found a spot in a bar to have a drink and take it all in. The interactions with the Sardinians at the end of our cycling days are the icing on the cake."

LAUREN HEFFERON founded Ciclismo Classico in 1988 with a dream to combine a passion for bicycling with her Italian roots, the visual arts, and outdoor education. Director and CEB (Chief Executive Biker) Lauren drives all visionary aspects of Ciclismo Classico, from itinerary design and tour leader training to marketing and company strategy. Life and politics revolve around two-wheeled activities for Lauren, who is a devoted cycling promoter. Commuting everywhere by bike, she supports cycling causes, such as Rails-to-Trails, Bikes Belong, Pan-Mass Challenge, and MassBike.

If You Go

▶ **Getting There:** Rides begin in the Alghero region, which is served from Rome and Milan by Alitalia (800-223-5730; www.alitalia.com).
▶ **Best Time to Visit:** Sardinia has a Mediterranean climate, with the warmest, driest weather from late spring through early fall. Earlier spring and later fall will be a bit cooler.
▶ **Guides/Outfitters:** Ciclismo Classico (800-866-7314; www.ciclismoclassico.com) leads several tours of Sardinia.
▶ **Level of Difficulty:** This trip covers 152 miles (245 km) over five days of riding. It's rated easy.
▶ **Accommodations:** Visit Sardegna.com to view lodging options.

DESTINATION 23

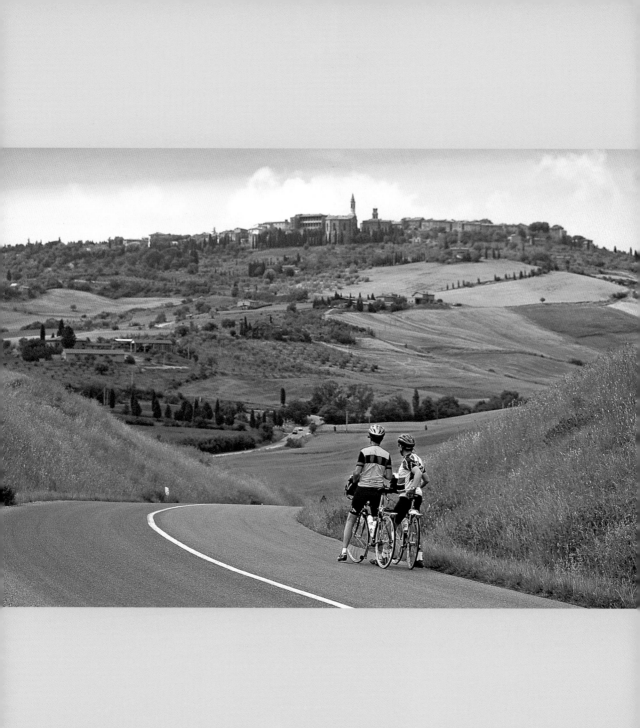

TUSCANY

RECOMMENDED BY **Tania Worgull**

Many connoisseurs of Italy will tell you that the soul of the country is found among the small hill towns and farms of rural Tuscany—though it's a soul that can only be understood by travelers who linger. Taking in Tuscany by bike is the perfect way to experience this picture-book countryside of millennia-old castles, orchards of olive and fig trees, and endless vineyards—and an ideal justification for partaking of its many gastronomic charms.

"There's no question that the riding is beautiful," Tania Worgull began. "There are spectacular winding, rolling roads, and the scenery is gorgeous. The contrast between southern Tuscany and the Chianti region is tremendous. The south has more rolling pastures, with expansive views and sheep-dotted hills; Chianti is more heavily wooded with forests of pine, oak, cork, and chestnut trees, and vineyards nestled here and there. The colors are so vibrant—vivid greens and bright red poppies in the spring, wonderfully muted olives and browns in the fall. It's no wonder so many photographers and painters come here to try and capture the many iconic scenes Tuscany offers. Guests often mention that the riding is more challenging than they imagined, hillier, but within reach for less-seasoned riders. But a cycling tour of Tuscany goes beyond what you experience in the saddle. There's great food to fuel you, fine local wines (many of which you may not find outside of the region) at the end of the ride, and of course, the warmth of the Tuscan people."

One cannot hope to traverse all of Tuscany in the course of an average cycling excursion. So Tania shared a few of her regular stops. One is Castellina in Chianti, a medieval town situated on a ridge astride the valleys of the Arbia, Elsa, and Pesa Rivers. Like many villages in the area, Castellina in Chianti has Etruscan and Roman roots, and remnants

OPPOSITE:
The cycling
through Tuscany
is just hilly
enough to
justify extrahearty
meals.

24

DESTINATION

of both cultures rest side by side. Preferred lodging here is Palazzo Squarcialupi, a fourteenth-century palace with sweeping hillside views. A memorable ride from Castellina in Chianti takes you to the formidable grounds of Castello di Brolio, the birthplace of Chianti wine. "You climb high above the vineyards," Tania continued, "and as you proceed along the ridge, you get a 360-degree view of the countryside. If the wind is right, you may hear sheep bells tinkling in the distance. Soon you descend through several tiny hamlets and Castello di Brolio appears, high on a hill." The castle (in one form or another) has been in Ricasoli hands since 1141, and the family is credited with creating the blend that we now know as Chianti Classico. (The original blend, created by Bettino Ricasoli in 1872, consisted of 70 percent Sangiovese, 15 percent Malvasia Bianca, and 15 percent Canaiolo grapes. Today, any blend with at least 80 percent Sangiovese grapes can be legally classified as Chianti Classico.)

Another Tuscan "must" for oenophiles is a visit to the walled village of Montalcino, home of one of the region's finest wines, Brunello di Montalcino. Riding from San Quirico, you climb above the Val d'Orcia region, with rolling hills dotted with vineyards and stately cypresses. You'll pass the Abbazia di Sant'Antimo, an active abbey that dates back to the twelfth century; depending on when you pass, you may hear the resident brothers sing Gregorian chants. A little farther along Montalcino comes into view—a vast fourteenth-century fortified hill town dominating the landscape. The Brunello grape (called Sangiovese Grosso) is a variant of the Sangiovese, yet the final product is quite different, as wine blogger "Iron" Chevsky has explained: "Brunello di Montalcino, of course, is normally bigger than Chianti in every respect—having more complex fruit, bigger tannin, greater balance, more supple texture."

"When I've introduced new visitors to Tuscany, one aspect of the trip that stands out for them is—not surprisingly—the food," Tania said. "I have several favorites. One is the bruschetta that's served in the town of Radda at a place called Bar Dante Alighieri Di Ferrucci Fabrizio. It has to be the best bruschetta in the world—just the right amount of garlic and salt, and the tomatoes are unlike any I've ever had. Another is the pecorino cheese in the town of Pienza. It's a hard cheese made from sheep's milk. As you walk around in Pienza, the aroma is amazing, and you can look over the back of the wall that lines the city and see the sheep grazing in the pastures beyond. In Gaiole in Chianti, I've taken a private cooking class at a farm where you learn how to make fresh pasta and accompanying sauces. Even the gelato you can find at many stands along the road is memorable."

DESTINATION 24

Whether it's a walk along a cobblestoned street in an ancient walled city while vendors hawk fresh produce, or a sunset savored from the deck of a castle-turned-hotel as you sip a fine Brunello, Tuscany will likely leave you with a few treasured memories. Tania recalled one special moment: "I was out riding by myself one morning, and I came upon a group of older Italian bicyclists, all men in their sixties and seventies. They were in their riding kits, and perhaps not in the best of shape—some bigger bellies were certainly visible. I began passing them, and they were giving me a jovial hard time. They called me what I interpreted as 'Skinny Legs,' though I think something was lost in translation. They welcomed me to finish my ride with them and showed the true Italian hospitality. They made me feel part of the local culture."

TANIA WORGULL is president of Trek Travel, a bike tour operator providing vacations of a lifetime from the seat of a bike. Tania has more than twenty years' experience in the active travel industry, has been with Trek Travel ten years, and has visited more than thirty countries. Her passion for cycling and travel drew her to the industry and guides the company's direction and strategy.

If You Go

▶ **Getting There:** The wonders of Tuscany are most easily reached via Florence.

▶ **Best Time to Visit:** Late spring and early fall provide pleasant temperatures; summers may be warm for some.

▶ **Guides/Outfitters:** Companies leading trips through Tuscany include Trek Travel (866-464-8735; www.trektravel.com) and VBT (800-245-3868; www.vbt.com).

▶ **Level of Difficulty:** This tour entails four full days of riding, averaging 40+ miles (65+ km) a day. It's rated moderate to difficult.

▶ **Accommodations:** Palazzo Squarcialupi (+39 0577 741186; www.palazzosquarcialupi .com) in Castellina in Chianti, Park Hotel Le Fonti (+39 0588 85219; www.parkhotelle fonti.com) in Volterra, Palazzo del Capitano (+39 0577 899 028; www.palazzodelcapitano .com) in San Quirico, and Castello di Spaltenna (+39 0577 749 483; www.spaltenna.it) in Spaltenna come well recommended.

BALTIC STATES

RECOMMENDED BY **Marius Mauragas**

"Many people arrive at the Baltic states with low expectations," Marius Mauragas led off. "Their preconception is that these are ex-Soviet satellite countries, so they must be derelict and very poor. When they disembark, they're very surprised. In the Baltic states— Lithuania, Latvia, and Estonia—nature and culture are nicely intertwined. The old town sections of our cities are comparable to many western European cities in terms of architecture and history, though perhaps not as large. You can see the influences of the West and the East combining. Our lakes, rivers, and forests are largely unspoiled; likewise, for our beaches. Guests have mentioned to me that you can smell the nature, the wildness of the place. We don't have mountains, so the terrain is easy to bike—you can ride as many miles as you wish. The best riding is along the Baltic Sea. When you're finished with the seaside ride, you can quickly transfer to one of the cities. Within a short time, you can experience very different sides of Baltic life. And since it's just 330 miles (530 km) from Vilnius in the south of Lithuania and Tallinn in the north of Estonia, you can experience three different cultures at a leisurely riding pace."

Lithuania, Latvia, and Estonia rest along the eastern shore of the Baltic Sea, tucked north of Poland and south of Finland, with Belarus and Russia looming to the east. The three small nations have periodically fallen under the sway of their larger neighbors— including Germany and Sweden—for much of modern history. The three states were under the control of Russia through much of the nineteenth century up until World War I, and then its successor, the Soviet Union, from the end of World War II until 1991. It's interesting to note that a 1989 protest called the Baltic Way, in which two million people created a human chain stretching from Tallinn to Vilnius, helped usher in the dissolution of the Soviet Union.

"The landscape of each of the countries is quite similar," Marius continued, "though the major cities have a different feeling. Vilnius has a baroque influence; Riga, Latvia, is more Germanic; Tallinn has a medieval feeling and was built by Scandinavians. Each country has a different language, though they are related and non-Slavic. I would say that the mentalities of the people are more or less the same. The food has a Germanic slant and tends to be on the heavier side. We have three main products—pork, potatoes, and beer—well, I joke. But historically, there are not a lot of vegetables grown here, though we import them now. Food—and for that matter, everything else—is very inexpensive by western standards. You can get 16 ounces (½ liter) of beer for one or two euros, a good meal for five to seven euros. The Baltics are still a good value, and the streets are very safe. You can walk at night everywhere with no problems."

Marius suggests beginning your travels in Vilnius, Lithuania's capital. The city sits astride the Neris River, in a valley between wooded hills and deep pine forests (30 percent of the Baltic states are forested). Here, you can walk winding streets that boast churches and monasteries of Gothic and baroque provenance. Brightly colored houses provide a festive atmosphere. A warm-up ride takes you to the town of Trakai and beside Lake Galve and its island castle, where the first king of Lithuania was crowned in 1253. Some of the best riding in Lithuania is along the Curonian Spit, a 60-mile (96-km) sand-dune peninsula that stretches between the Baltic and a lagoon along the country's southwest coast. Much of the spit is preserved as a national park, and is listed as a UNESCO World Heritage site. "There are small fishing villages along the spit, and Nida, which is a resort town. (Nida was the summer home of the German novelist Thomas Mann, and you can visit the site.) The beach at Nida is ranked among the top ten in all of Europe, though all the beaches along the spit are very clean. The water averages 65 degrees, so it's warm enough to swim in despite our northern latitude. Curonian Spit is also very green; many pines were planted in the nineteenth century to help prevent erosion, and the scent of pine mixes pleasantly with the sea air as you ride."

From the Lithuanian coast, you'll move north to Latvia and the capital of Riga, the largest city in the Baltic states. Though a thriving commercial center, Riga boasts a wonderfully preserved old town—Vecrīga—that dates back eight hundred years and was established as a trading settlement for German knights. It includes intact structures from the fifteenth and sixteenth centuries. One of Marius's favorite rides around Riga takes you out to the seaside resort area of Jurmala. "The sand here is very hard, and we can ride

DESTINATION

25

right on the beach," he said. "Along the beach, there's an interesting juxtaposition of peculiar wooden summer cottages, grand old villas, and opulent new constructions. This speaks to the intersection of the Baltics' past and present." Crossing into Estonia, you'll have a chance to cycle in Lahemaa National Park, the nation's first and largest preserve, a blend of coastal bluffs, dense forests, striking glacial boulders, millennia-old bogs, cascading waterfalls, and several manor houses. "In the time of the Russian empire, Lahemaa was tied to St. Petersburg, and some nobles had their retreats here," Marius explained. "One of the manors—Sagadi—can now accommodate guests. A visit to Lahemaa gives you a great blend of Baltic nature and culture, and captures what this trip is all about."

MARIUS MAURAGAS is based in Vilnius, Lithuania, and studied at Vilnius University. For many years, he has organized Baltics trips for Djoser. For two years, Marius served as president of Djoser's worldwide consortium of land agents, responsible for ensuring the quality and Djoser philosophy of "active adventures with freedom." In addition to the Baltics biking programs, Marius organizes cultural tours to the region.

DESTINATION

25

If You Go

▶ **Getting There:** Trips usually begin in Vilnius, Lithuania, which is served by a number of airlines including Lufthansa (800-645-3880; www.lufthansa.com) from Frankfurt, and Ryanair (+44 871 246 0002; www.ryanair.com) from London. Lufthansa and Ryanair also serve Tallinn, Estonia, where excursions end.

▶ **Best Time to Visit:** May to September offers the most consistent weather.

▶ **Guides/Outfitters:** Djoser USA (877-356-7376; www.djoserusa.com) leads bike tours through the Baltic states.

▶ **Level of Difficulty:** This tour involves six days of riding of between 15 and 25 miles (24 to 40 km) a day. It's rated easy to moderate.

▶ **Accommodations:** Lodging options in Lithuania are highlighted at www.lithuania-tourism.co.uk; in Latvia, at www.latvia.travel/en; in Estonia, Sagadi Manor (+372 676 7888; www.sagadi.ee) comes well recommended.

CASCO BAY REGION

RECOMMENDED BY **Steve Fuller**

Some great bike rides can be found several plane rides and many time zones away. Others may be right in your own backyard . . . especially if you live in the Casco Bay region of Maine. "I've biked in many more glamorous places, but I think the area around Freeport has some of the best road biking you'll find anywhere, period," Steve Fuller declared. "You have the proximity of the ocean, some good climbs, decent roads, remarkably little traffic, and the vibrant coastal towns of Brunswick and Freeport. There's an incredible feeling you get riding along a coastal meadow when the three o'clock cooler breeze kicks up."

The greater Casco Bay region—from the city of Portland in the south to Brunswick in the north—brings many of Maine's best facets together in one place. It's here that the sandy beaches that characterize the southern part of the Pine Tree State's shoreline meet the rock-ribbed, cove-laden coast that's conjured up by the phrase "Downeast Maine." Summer visitors can easily shadow a lobsterman in the morning and bodysurf on a pleasant beach in the afternoon. The city of Portland—consistently ranked one of the best places to live in the United States—has a thriving restaurant and music scene that belies its modest population. Within a short cycle from Portland or Freeport, you can take in lighthouses, forts, and captains' homes that speak to Maine's seafaring history.

Mention Freeport and anyone with a mailbox may recall a little mail-order house that calls this seaside town home. L.L.Bean was established after its namesake—Leon Leonwood Bean—created a shoe that combined a rubber boot sole with a leather upper. In 1912, he obtained a mailing list of nonresident Maine hunting license holders and sent out a flyer promoting his "Maine Hunting Shoe," with a money-back guarantee. Ninety of the first one hundred pairs sold were returned, but Bean kept his word . . . and the original design flaw was fixed. The rest, as they say, is history. Today, more than 200 million

121

catalogs are sent out to customers around the world annually, and the flagship store in the middle of downtown Freeport (marked by a 15-foot-tall Maine Hunting Shoe) remains open twenty-four hours a day, 365 days a year; the policy stems from Mr. Bean's commitment to serve hunters and fisherman keeping very early or very late hours.

It so happens that one of Steve's favorite rides departs from the front steps of the retail store. "The route heads south to Casco Bay and then follows the shoreline in a northeasterly direction to the town of Brunswick," Steve continued. "You'll pass through the Pennellville district [home of several fine mansions built by the shipbuilding Pennell family in the eighteenth and nineteenth centuries] and along some coastal meadows until you come into the town proper. I think that Brunswick may be one of the most underappreciated towns in Maine. It has fantastic coffee shops like Little Dog and some of the best record stores (Vinylhaven and Bull Moose) in New England—thanks at least in part to the presence of Bowdoin College." Bowdoin gives Brunswick a burst of intellectual vigor you might not expect in an otherwise quiet coastal town.

"After a stop in Brunswick for an espresso or ice cream, I like to cut inland toward the village of New Gloucester," Steve said. "There are some nice climbs as you move from the coast. My destination is a place called Pineland Farms. For almost one hundred years, Pineland served as a home for Maine's mentally handicapped. When it closed in 1996, there were twenty-eight buildings on 1,600 acres. The campus became derelict, but in 2000 it was purchased by the Libra Foundation [a philanthropic entity] and rehabilitated. Today it's a 5,000-acre working farm, where organic produce and beef are raised and artisan cheese is made. From Pineland, I'll head back in a southeasterly direction toward Yarmouth and South Freeport. In South Freeport, a visit to Town Landing Harbor is a must. It's a picturesque little village enclave that looks out on Harraseeket Bay. I'd recommend grabbing lunch or early dinner at the Harraseeket Lunch & Lobster Company. You can watch the fishing boats come in with their catch, tie on a bib, and tuck into a fresh lobster." In 2010, more than 93 million pounds of lobster were harvested from Maine waters. Plated *Homarus americanus* can take infinite forms, but the locals prefer it simple—steamed in the shell, with sides of melted butter and lemon.

The ride Steve described is one of many options in greater Casco Bay. Another popular tour will take you around one (or several) of the islands served by Casco Bay's fleet of ferries—Peaks Island, Little Diamond Island, Great Diamond Island, Diamond Cove, Long Island, Chebeague Island, Cousins Island, and Cliff Island. Another idea is to cycle

OPPOSITE:
Rides along Casco Bay can take you past a number of lighthouses, including Portland Head Light in Cape Elizabeth.

DESTINATION

26

to some of the region's lighthouses, including Portland Head Light (which dates back to 1791) and the lighthouse at Two Lights State Park, which was immortalized in Edward Hopper's *The Lighthouse at Two Lights.*

STEVE FULLER is the chief marketing officer for L.L.Bean Inc. He oversees all strategic marketing functions for the company including advertising, customer planning, and Web presence. Most recently he has been asked to oversee L.L.Bean's international business, including its move into China. Steve played a key role in the development of Bean's Outdoor Advantage Program, the company's co-branded Visa card, which he helped to grow into one of the largest affinity programs in the country. He also was responsible for the establishment of Bean's relationship with Subaru and the development of the auto-maker's L.L.Bean editions in the United States and Japan. Steve has been on the boards of several environmental and outdoor organizations, including the New England Nordic Ski Association, Friends of Casco Bay, and the Appalachian Mountain Club. An avid cyclist, Steve has ridden throughout the United States and in Europe.

DESTINATION

26

If You Go

▶ **Getting There:** Visitors fly into Portland, which is served by many carriers, including Delta (800-221-1212; www.delta.com) and United Airlines (800-864-8331; www.united.com).

▶ **Best Time to Visit:** Weather is fairly reliable from mid-May and mid-October.

▶ **Guides/Outfitters:** Summer Feet Cycling Adventures (866-857-9544; www.summerfeet.net) offers tours of greater Portland, including island and lighthouse rides. You'll find great resources for planning your own trip at www.exploremaine.org/bike.

▶ **Level of Difficulty:** You'll want to have at least three days to experience Casco Bay by bike. Riding difficulty is rated moderate.

▶ **Accommodations:** Two popular properties in Freeport are Harraseeket Inn (800-342-6423; www.harraseeketinn.com) and Applewood Inn B&B (877-954-1358; www.applewoodusa.com). Visit Portland (207-772-5800; www.visitportland.com) lists accommodations in the city.

LEELANAU PENINSULA

RECOMMENDED BY **Tim Meyer**

"For a great family bike trip, it's pretty hard to beat Michigan's Leelanau Peninsula," Tim Meyer asserted. "The scenery is constantly spectacular; the whole area is absent of 'gotta ride through this to get to that' stretches, which is say, every part is worth riding. There are overnight spots nicely spaced along the route, with your choice of motels or camp-grounds; you never have to go more than 20 or 30 miles (32 to 48 km) to find a place to stay. There are lots of lakes up on the peninsula—Lake Michigan among them—with crystal-clear water. The inland lakes are 70 degrees; Lake Michigan is a little cooler, but certainly swimmable in the summer. Much of Sleeping Bear Dunes National Lakeshore rests on the peninsula, and you can ferry out to North Manitou and South Manitou Islands, which are also part of the preserve. (Sleeping Bear Dunes was voted the most beautiful area in the United States by the viewers of ABC's *Good Morning America* in 2011.) When our kids were born, they spent their first summers being towed around the Leelanau in a Burley trailer by my wife and me. Now, twenty-four years later, our eldest son, Matt, is running one of our bike shops, and the younger boy, Ried, is studying wil-derness adventure education at Green Mountain College. I like to think that those early times on the Leelanau Peninsula helped give them an appreciation of the outdoors."

The Leelanau Peninsula juts north from Traverse City along the eastern shores of Lake Michigan. Tim likes to begin his rides from Traverse City, which is frequently named one of the top ten places to retire in the United States, thanks in part to its proximity to first-rate outdoor amenities, like the TART (Traverse Area Recreation & Transportation Trails), a bike trail system. "From Traverse City, you can head north to the Old Mission Peninsula," Tim continued, "maybe visiting some of the eighteen wineries along the way. You head up along the east arm along Lake Michigan's Grand Traverse Bay and back down along the west arm. It's a 35- or 40-mile (56- to 64-km) loop back to Traverse City, a great warm-up before starting up the Leelanau Peninsula." One may not think of great wine when northern Michigan comes to mind, but the Old Mission Peninsula rests close to the 45th parallel, a latitude known for its superior grapes. This is Riesling country; some grapes are left on the vine until late fall, when they are harvested for ice wine.

After another night in Traverse City, you'll start up the Leelanau on the peninsula's east side. You'll ride through the resort area of Suttons Bay and Fountain Point House, where a gusher of sparkling water has flowed since 1867 (the result of an unsuccessful oil exploration). Northport is the next town, the last on the peninsula. "You could get a motel room in Northport," Tim said, "but I like to head a few miles farther north to Leelanau State Park. This is an outstanding camping spot. You can go right to the tip of the pinkie of lower Michigan at Lighthouse Point. The lighthouse here was built in 1858 and now is preserved as a museum. After a night at the park, you cycle down the other side of the pinkie to the fishing village of Leland. From Leland, you have the option to take a ferry out to the Manitou Islands, which are 16 and 18 miles offshore." North and South Manitou Islands are part of Sleeping Bear Dunes National Lakeshore; South Manitou may be familiar to some for the 100-foot lighthouse (established in 1871) that marks its natural harbor, a safe haven for steamers plying Lake Michigan between Chicago and Michigan's Upper Peninsula. "Sometimes we'll leave our bikes in Leland and take backpacks out to the islands to camp overnight," Tim added. "There are several rustic campsites on South Manitou, and wilderness camping on North Manitou. From South Manitou, you can see a shipwreck (the Liberian freighter *Francisco Morazan*, which went down in 1960)."

Returning to the mainland at Leland, you'll ride to the southwest and roll into Sleeping Bear Dunes National Lakeshore proper. The reserve extends some 35 miles along the coast and showcases immense sand dunes perched atop towering headlands, handiwork of steady winds from the west and glacial movement; some dunes, including Sleeping Bear itself, tower 400 feet above Lake Michigan. "There are several lakes and rivers in Sleeping Bear Dunes," Tim continued, "including Little Glen and Big Glen Lakes, which were once connected to Lake Michigan. You can rent a canoe and paddle along the lake and the adjoining Crystal River and make out the successive shorelines as the lake was formed. There's a little town called Glen Arbor nearby, one of the most outstanding little places on the planet, with quaint little restaurants, bed-and-breakfasts, and a great bar— Art's Tavern—that has a pool table that can be lowered down into a hatch in the floor to make room for more tables or dancing. While you're visiting, you'll also want to do the Dune Climb; a lot of people like to roll down after they've trudged up.

"One must-do ride at Sleeping Bear Dunes takes you up to Inspiration Point, on the south side of Big Glen Lake. The road climbs and winds, winds and climbs, and though it's not terrifically long, it's a significant uphill. You don't get the view until you reach the very top, but it's worth the wait and the work. From the overlook, you can see Big Glen Lake, the Crystal River, the town of Glen Arbor, the Dune Climb to the south, and out across Lake Michigan to the Manitou Islands."

TIM MEYER grew up in Ohio riding his bike to get to school, deliver papers, and to tow a lawn mower to neighbors' yards. His first big bike trip was TOSRV, Tour of the Scioto River Valley, with high school friends. He cycled across the United States with Bikecentennial '76 at the age of nineteen. Just after moving to Holland, Michigan, as newlyweds, he and his wife, Lydia, rode to the Mackinac Bridge and back, discovering the natural wonder of the Lake Michigan coast. Tim opened Rock 'n Road Cycle (www.rockn roadcycle.com) in Grand Haven, Michigan, and with his son Matt operates bicycle stores there and in Holland. Both Tim and Lydia have worked with Adventure Cycling Association (as Bikecentennial '76 is now known) to lead and develop rides in Michigan. They have toured extensively in the United States together and with their children.

If You Go

▶ **Getting There:** Trips begin in Traverse City, which is served by American Eagle (800-433-7300; www.aa.com) and Delta (800-221-1212; www.delta.com).

▶ **Best Time to Visit:** You'll find the most consistent weather from June through September.

▶ **Guides/Outfitters:** Adventure Cycling (800-755-2453; www.adventurecycling.org) has assembled tours in the Leelanau region. Brick Wheels (231-947-4274; www.brickwheels .com) can also provide guidance.

▶ **Level of Difficulty:** Easy to moderate, with an average of 25 miles (40 km) a day.

▶ **Accommodations:** Leelanau Communications (www.leelanau.com) lists lodging options on the Leelanau Peninsula.

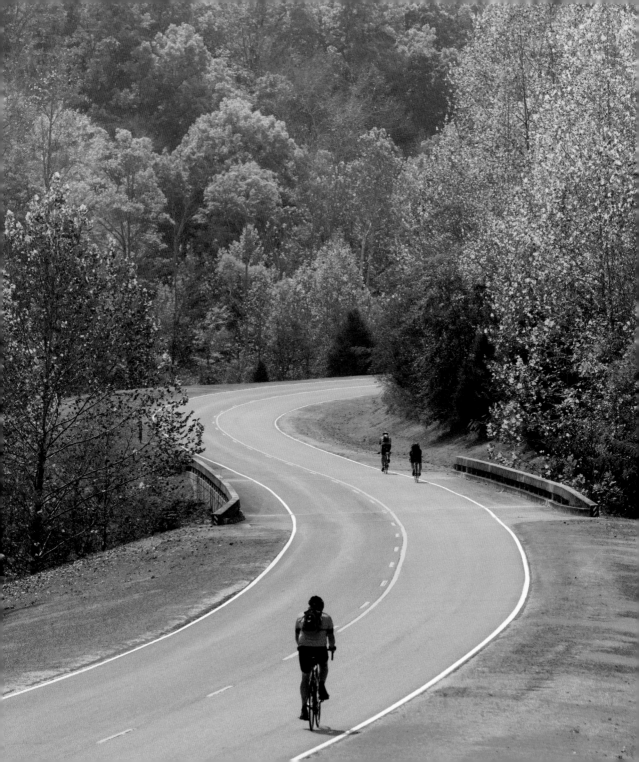

NATCHEZ TRACE

RECOMMENDED BY **Paul Wood**

"The Natchez Trace is an amazing ride that most people just haven't heard about," Paul Wood of Black Bear Adventure Bicycle Tours began. "It has all the attributes that cyclists enjoy—a quiet, smooth road that stretches hundreds of miles; a diversity of terrain, from the lowlands of the Mississippi Delta to long, rolling, twisting terrain in the north along the edge of the Appalachians; and no commercial activity—neither trucks nor billboards—to interrupt the flow of your day. The trace can be geared toward all levels of cyclists. You don't have to worry about navigating; every mile is marked. If you want to get in big miles, you certainly can do so. Or you can choose to take it slow and immerse yourself in southern culture and antebellum history. Between the plantations and Civil War battle sites, there's so much of the American South's past associated with the road."

The Natchez Trace stretches 444 miles (715 km), from the city of Natchez near the southwestern corner of Mississippi to Nashville, Tennessee. Along the way, it passes the length of Mississippi (through Jackson and Tupelo), through a swatch of Alabama (the shoals region), and on north through south central Tennessee, passing the town of Franklin before reaching Nashville. Though bikes are a fairly recent addition to the trace, humans have been using this north-south route for thousands of years . . . and animals for perhaps ten thousand. It was trod first by members of the Choctaw, Natchez, and Chickasaw tribes, then French and Spanish settlers; in the early nineteenth century, it was heavily used by boatmen from the Ohio River valley. These boatmen—known as "Kaintucks"—would float goods down the Ohio to the Mississippi and farther south to Natchez or New Orleans. Once their merchandise was sold, they'd dismantle their flatboats, sell the wood, and begin their journey home on foot or by horseback, generally going through Nashville toward points north and east. The advent of steamship travel

OPPOSITE:
Very flat in its southern reaches, the Natchez Trace gets hillier as it moves through Tennessee.

DESTINATION

28

made the Kaintucks' one-way journey less practical, and the development of other roads made the Natchez Trace less significant, yet it was still used by postmen and by soldiers during the Civil War. The National Park Service recognized the trace's historic value and took the road under its care in 1937. Over the next seventy years, the Park Service slowly transformed the trace into a parkway; work was finished in 2005, and the Natchez Trace is now recognized as a National Scenic Byway.

Paul likes to begin at the southern end of the parkway and make his way north. "I try to leave a day or two at the start of the ride to enjoy Natchez," he continued. "It's a fun town, and there are some beautiful antebellum structures that symbolize the legacy of the cotton barons—Dunleith and Monmouth Plantations come to mind. There's also great blues music in the pubs—you're in Delta country, after all. Moving north toward Jackson on the first day of riding, we stop at the Emerald Mound archaeological site. The Indian tribes that lived in this region were for the most part mound dwellers. There are other mounds along the route, but this is the best example. The road is mostly flat, and I usually get all the way to Jackson in one day, which is about 100 miles (160 km). If you have the energy—or the time—it's worthwhile to ride over to Vicksburg (or later on, Shiloh in Tennessee) to visit the battlefield. Whether you tour the site on your own or with a guide, it's not hard to envision the sights/sounds/smells of battle when you're in such proximity to a spot where so many died (casualties at Vicksburg were in excess of 20,000 men). You ride away with a sense of the horror of the Civil War and the terrible atrocities that man can commit upon himself."

Two more fairly long days in the saddle (80 and 85 miles [128 and 137 km], respectively) bring you to Tupelo, Mississippi. "Tupelo is a favorite stop along the ride for me," Paul said. "Up until this point, you've been immersed in what I'd describe as antebellum culture. In Tupelo, you feel a city that's more modern. Of course, it's also the birthplace of Elvis Presley, and fans can make the pilgrimage to his childhood home. As you leave Mississippi, you cross the Tennessee River and start to come into rolling hills in the brief section of Alabama the parkway crosses. There's a rest day in Florence, Alabama, at a lovely Marriott resort, and then we cross into Tennessee. I have to say that the Tennessee stretch is one of my favorite riding spots anywhere. The road here—a twisty, undulating path through beautiful countryside, with horse farms and forests—is spectacular. One great stop along this stretch of the ride is in the little town of Leiper's Fork, just outside Franklin. There's a general store there that serves classic southern cuisine, including fried chicken, collard greens, black-eyed peas, mac 'n cheese, and of course, homemade corn bread. After dinner, they clear the tables, push them to the side, and bring some local musicians out. The music could be bluegrass, old-timey country, or more modern country. Whatever they're playing, it's a real taste of Tennessee."

PAUL WOOD has ridden bikes as long as he can remember, and has always been passionate about the simple pleasure of riding a bike. A competitive cyclist through the late eighties and nineties, he started Black Bear Adventure Bicycle Tours in 2003 with the vision of showing the world the incredible cycling and natural beauty the South has to offer. Paul first designed tours along the Blue Ridge and Natchez Trace Parkways and now offers tours in many of the country's most desirable cycling destinations. "A good friend once told me that marrying your vocation with your avocation is the key to success," Paul said, "and I have been lucky enough to do just that."

If You Go

▶ **Getting There:** The trace's southern terminus is in Natchez, Mississippi. The closest commercial airport is in Alexandria, Louisiana, which is served by Continental (800-523-3273; www.continental.com) and Delta (800-221-1212; www.delta.com). The northern terminus is Nashville, which is served by many carriers.

▶ **Best Time to Visit:** Visitors will find more moderate temperatures from late winter to mid spring and again through the fall.

▶ **Guides/Outfitters:** Black Bear Adventure Bicycle Tours (888-339-8687; www.blackbearadventures.com) leads tours on the Natchez Trace. The National Park Service (www.nps.gov/natr) provides extensive resources for cyclists.

▶ **Level of Difficulty:** You'll cover 444 miles (715 km) over seven days of riding. It's rated moderate to difficult.

▶ **Accommodations:** The Natchez Trace Compact website (www.scenictrace.com) lists lodging options in communities along the trace.

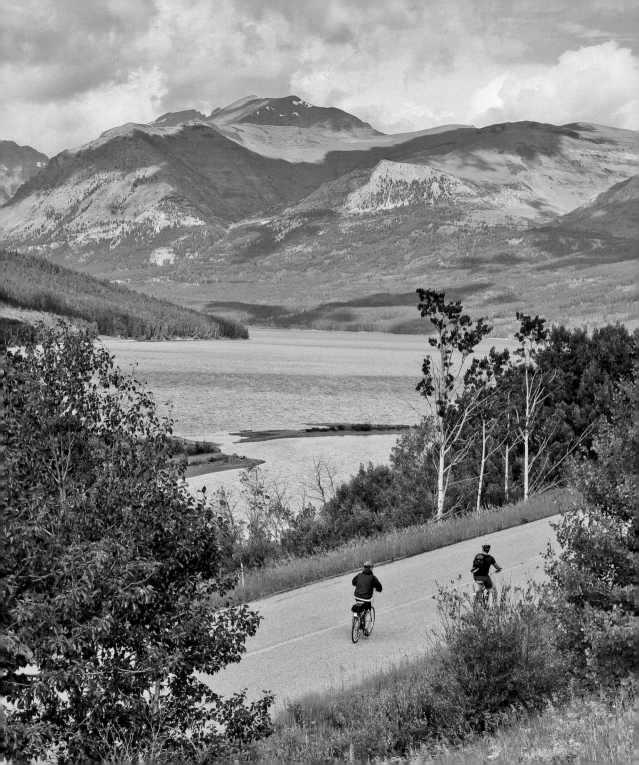

GLACIER/WATERTON LAKES
NATIONAL PARKS

RECOMMENDED BY **Linden Bader**

"Glacier and Waterton Lakes National Parks are among the most stunningly beautiful places on earth," Linden Bader declared. "The scenery is breathtaking, as you move from a temperate rain forest to an arid alpine setting and back, and there's always the chance that you'll come upon wildlife. Add to this the sense of triumph you can experience as you make it up over one of the world's most famous routes, Going-to-the-Sun Road, and you have a trip that's almost beyond words."

Glacier National Park comprises more than one million acres in northwestern Montana, just to the northeast of the growing recreational region of Kalispell/Whitefish; the park abuts Alberta and contiguous Waterton Lakes National Park. Contrary to popular perception, the park is named not for existing glaciers (of which a few do remain), but for the work earlier glaciers did at the conclusion of the last ice age. These glaciers slowly scoured away deep valleys and sharp ridges, carving rugged mountains and deep lakes en route. Glacier's mountains are actually a southern extension of the Canadian Rockies, more sedimentary in composition than the granite-based American Rockies. The way these formations have worn away adds to their dramatic nature. Glacier is also special because of its abundant animal life. Every big game animal that was here originally can still be found here—wolves, mountain lions, wolverines, lynx, and of course, grizzlies. The presence of these predators, especially the bears, intensifies one's senses.

There are many high points as you cycle around Glacier/Waterton Lakes National Parks. For most, the pinnacle is conquering Going-to-the-Sun Road. Completed in 1933, Going-to-the-Sun Road has the special distinction of being the only American roadway designated both as a National Historic Landmark and a National Historic Civil Engineering Landmark. It was one of the first National Park Service projects conceived

OPPOSITE:
Cyclists roll along
Two Medicine
Lake in the
southeastern
section of
Glacier
National
Park.

DESTINATION

29

133

for both automobiles and bicycles. Going-to-the-Sun Road—which is named for a mountain in the park, not for its generally easterly direction—highlights many of the park's totem characteristics, from glacial lakes to waterfalls to old-growth forests to windswept passes, as it parallels the Continental Divide. Linden described the experience in its entirety. "You start out early from Lake McDonald Lodge, as park rules dictate that you need to be at the top of Logan Pass (6,646 feet), which is 21 miles (33 km), by 11 a.m. Leaving the lake, you begin with 10 miles (16 km) of flat, shaded riding; here, you're still in the rain forest section of the park. It's very quiet, no one else is out, and it's a perfect way to get your wheels spinning. You'll soon come to Logan Creek, which runs down from Logan Pass. From here you get a view up to where you'll be going (some 3,000 feet in elevation gain). You're still in the forest at this point, though the next 3 miles (5 km) are steep, a 7 percent grade. You emerge from the forest at McDonald Creek, where you get a view of Heaven's Peak (8,987 feet). At a spot called 'The Loop,' the grade decreases a bit, but you still have 10 miles (16 km) to go. Soon you'll reach the Garden Wall, the immense vertical rock face that the road was carved into. The flowers can be spectacular here, though the drop-off to the valley on the right is thousands of feet—not for someone with acrophobia. After a few more bends you'll see Logan Pass. The last mile gets steep again, and you enter the Krummholz Zone, where the trees are stunted because of the wind and cold. It's here that you'll often see mountain goats.

"When you reach the pass, you're at the Continental Divide. There's a sign that you can have your picture taken next to. I think everyone who does it has a huge feeling of accomplishment. Some people can make it in two hours; others it takes right up to eleven o'clock. When you tell people who drove up to Logan Pass that you just rode up there, they can't believe it. After a little celebrating, you have 13 miles (20 km) of exhilarating downhill riding. I usually add a layer for that. When you reach St. Mary, there's a great little pie shop that also has huckleberry milkshakes. After a sweet treat, you have another 20 miles (32 km), some along the shores of Upper and Lower St. Mary Lakes, to the Many Glacier Hotel. As you ride in, you're looking at the eastern side of the Garden Wall—you've made a full circle! You almost always end with a headwind, which can be a little brutal. But once you get to the hotel, you can grab a beer from the bar, find a seat on the back deck of the hotel, and look out as the sun sets behind Mount Grinnell. Sometimes you'll see bears foraging on the hillside. This is one of my favorite places in the world."

Though Going-to-the-Sun is behind you, there's still some fine riding ahead as you move north to Waterton Lakes National Park. "Leaving Many Glacier Valley, you come into rangeland and may see hundreds of head of cattle," Linden described. "Real 'Big Sky' country. We then head up to Chief Mountain Overlook, 5 miles (8 km) of 6 percent grade. Chief Mountain rises by itself from the pastureland, something like a squared-off Devils Tower. Soon after, you cross the border, which is fun to do on a bicycle; you're still questioned about possessing firearms and produce, and you have to show your passport. Then you're climbing again, up to the Waterton Overlook. You can see across the three Waterton Lakes, and in the distance, the Prince of Wales Hotel, perched on a glacial moraine above the water like something out of a storybook. It's 10 more miles (16 km) to the hotel, which is said to be the windiest place in Canada; the hotel is cabled in place. We spend two nights at Prince of Wales. On the layover day, you can opt to do a hike, go canoeing or horseback riding, or bike to Cameron Lake and Red Rock Canyon. Here, you have a very good chance of seeing either grizzly or black bears."

Heading back into the United States the following day, you have the option of notching a century. "This is one of my favorite days on the trip," Linden continued. "We retrace part of our route from a few days before. After you pass the community of St. Mary (east of the lakes), be sure to look to the right to spot Fusillade Mountain. It was used in *The Chronicles of Narnia* movie; the Ice Queen's palace was digitally inserted into the mountainside! From here, you come into rolling terrain before a big climb to Looking Glass Pass. At the top, you start getting views of Medicine Lake and Two Medicine Valley—a very special spot. There's a funny optical illusion that occurs on this stretch. As you approach the valley, it seems as if you're going downhill, though you're still pedaling. As they leave the valley, riders have the sense that they're going up. I have to assure them that they're going downhill. You can sail the last 4 miles (6.5 km) right into East Glacier and Glacier Park Lodge. Thus far, you've gone 92 miles (148 km). We can send you on a 4-mile down-and-back so you can finish your century."

LINDEN BADER has been trip leader with Backroads since 2005. A San Francisco native and UC Berkeley grad, she left behind a career in the fashion industry to become a trip leader. Linden has traveled throughout Asia, Europe, and the Americas, and loves leading trips anywhere there are mountains. She believes there's no better way to connect with a place than by slowing down to a biking or walking pace.

DESTINATION

29

If You Go

▶ **Getting There:** Visitors can fly to Kalispell (25 miles [40 km] west of the park head-quarters), which is served by Alaska Airlines (800-252-7522; www.alaskaair.com) and United (800-864-8331; www.united.com). There's also Amtrak service to Glacier (800-872-7245; www.amtrak.com).

▶ **Best Time to Visit:** Peak biking season is June through September; October can be beautiful, but winter weather can blow in at any time. The Glacier National Park website (www.nps.gov/glac) lists conditions.

▶ **Guides/Outfitters:** Many tour companies lead trips through Glacier National Park, including Backroads (800-462-2848; www.backroads.com).

▶ **Level of Difficulty:** The trip above entails a minimum of 30 to 40 miles (48 to 64 km) a day for four days. It's rated moderate to difficult.

▶ **Accommodations:** In addition to many campgrounds, there are a number of lodging options inside Glacier National Park, including Lake McDonald Lodge; all are highlighted on the park's website (www.nps.gov/glac). Lodge reservations for Lake McDonald, Many Glacier Hotel, and Prince of Wales Hotel in Waterton can be made through Glacier Park, Inc. (406-892-2525; www.glacierparkinc.com).

THE NORTH

RECOMMENDED BY **Desiree Janssen**

Fields of wildly colored tulips, idyllic (and very practical) windmills peppered along a patchwork of dikes and canals, and one of the world's most bike-friendly cultures. All these elements—not to mention some wonderful pancakes and endless stretches of flatness—make the Netherlands a popular destination for biking enthusiasts. When Netherlands native Desiree Janssen set out to create a tour, she chose a path that would highlight the iconic elements of the Dutch way of life. "The Netherlands is a small country," she began, "just 150 kilometers (93 miles) by 300 kilometers (186 miles). Yet despite its small size, the twelve provinces are very different. I grew up in the southern part of the country. When I first visited the north I thought, 'This is the country I live in? It's the Holland that's in the picture books!' So our ride focuses on the provinces of Noord-Holland, Friesland, and Drenthe.

"Some people in the United States think of biking as something you go out and do," she added. "You wear different clothing, different shoes. In Netherlands, we don't re-dress when we're riding a bike. We wear what we wear. Biking is part of everyday life. Parents ride bikes with small children in front and back. I carry my groceries on my bike; I even carried a Christmas tree once! At traffic lights, there's a separate line for bicycles—bikes can go in front of the car, so you don't wait in exhaust fumes. Cyclists have a traffic light that lets them go first."

Tulips are in bloom in late April in the Netherlands, and it's a special time to ride—though the weather can be a little uncertain. "We have a saying about April," Desiree continued. "April has a mind of its own. It can sometimes be like summer, sometimes like winter. The first year I led the tour in 1999, it was almost freezing out, but since then, we've had beautiful weather—at least by Dutch standards. Though the tulips are

137

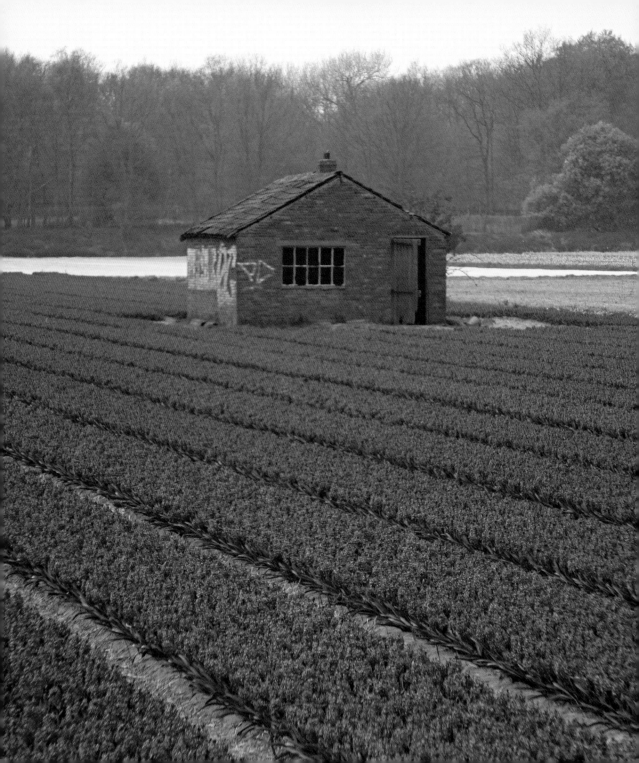

something to behold with your eyes, it's the smell of the hyacinth fields that make the biking spectacular. They literally take your breath away." Desiree begins her ride near one of the centerpieces of the Netherlands' tulip industry, in the city of Haarlem. One of her favorite rides departs from here. "Haarlem is close to the coast, and there's a two-way bike path that takes you out to the beach and through a long stretch of dunes," she described. "You know you're close to the water, but the dunes are in between, though now and then there's an opening to the beach. You can make a stop to see the beach. If you stick your feet in the water, you'll find it's cold! When you leave the dunes, you're close to the Keukenhof, a 79-acre park that showcases the work of bulb growers—the better the display they do, the more bulbs they'll sell. (More than 4.5 million tulips in one hundred varieties are on display!) As we loop back to Haarlem, we pass by fields where many bulbs are grown. As soon as the bulbs start blossoming, the flowers are cut so that the bulbs retain their vitality. Because the flowers would otherwise be wasted, many Dutch towns have *Bloemencorsos*—flower festivals. If you're lucky, you might visit Haarlem (or another town) during its annual flower parade, where incredible floats made of brightly colored flowers are feted through the street." (The beauty of the tulips can be almost maddening, and indeed, a certain madness surrounded the introduction of tulips in the 1630s, when "tulip mania" gripped Holland. The flowers became the focus of speculation, with single bulbs commanding multiples of a skilled workman's annual wages. Not surprisingly, the tulip bubble soon burst.)

As you may recall from elementary school geography classes, the Netherlands is an extremely low-lying country. Nearly 25 percent of the country actually rests under sea level. That's where the Netherlands' ingenious system of dikes and canals—and the pumping system *once* powered by windmills—comes to the rescue. Moving from Haarlem to Noord-Holland, you'll get a close-up look at the workings of the region's water control systems. "In 1928, many of the pump systems that were once powered by wind shifted to electricity," Desiree continued, "but in this region, eleven are still wind-power generated. The technology was very sophisticated for its time, and I like to visit one of the working windmills that's now operated as a museum, the Schermemolen. It provides a great explanation of how the windmills worked. During this portion of the tour, we ride at times along the top of dikes (levees). When you're on top of a dike, you're just a bit raised above the rest of the landscape—especially in the Netherlands. You're at roof level, and it gives you a very different perspective. You feel like you're in a miniature

OPPOSITE:
A field of tulips,
just outside the
Keukenhof, a
79-acre park that
showcases the
work of Dutch
bulb growers.

DESTINATION

30

train landscape." To the east is IJsselmeer—which was once an extension of the North Sea called the Zuiderzee. "The towns here—Hoorn and Enkhuizen—used to be seafaring towns," Desiree explained, "though when the barrier dam called Afsluitdijk was built across the Zuiderzee, they were effectively closed off from the sea. Some of the land was drained of water and reclaimed for farming or cattle; these reclaimed areas are called *polders*."

After a night on the lake in Enkhuizen, you'll ferry across IJsselmeer to Friesland. You'll enjoy a day exploring quiet lanes along the east side of the lake, and then you'll bike on to Drenthe. A visit to the village of Giethoorn, known as the "Venice of the North," is a must. Though the canals may speak to Italy, the thatched houses and humpback bridges remind you that you're in the north. You'll continue on to the Kasteel de Havixhorst, a grand manor house dating from 1753. "Not only is the Havixhorst a beautiful hotel, but its grounds are also home to a number of storks, Netherlands' national bird," Desiree said. "A sanctuary was established here, and the birds—which had dwindled to a population of only nineteen breeding pairs in 1969—have thrived. There are 120 pairs now, and you can view the birds from very close." After a morning enjoying the storks, you can ride on to Orvelte, which is maintained as a "museum village," which showcases traditional Dutch living from the nineteenth century. A popular exhibit shows how wooden clogs are made.

In the town of Odoorn, you may wish to sample one of the Netherlands' national delicacies—the pancake. "When people think of pancakes, they usually think of breakfast," Desiree explained. "You can have a dessert pancake, but we think of them as more of a savory food, like a soft-dough pizza. They're often served with peppers, shrimp, or mushrooms. In larger towns like Haarlem you'll also find wonderful Indonesian food, which goes back to the colonial days. The flavors of the Spice Islands—clove, nutmeg, cinnamon, and cumin—have been very much incorporated into our food."

DESIREE JANSSEN was born and raised in the Netherlands, and practically grew up on a bicycle. After studying to be an arts and crafts teacher, she embarked on a five-month journey to Southeast Asia. By the time she returned, she realized traditional teaching was not a good match for her—so she became involved with a Dutch bike tour company. Today, she leads bicycle tours in Europe for Austin-Lehman Adventures in the warmer months, and in the off-season works as an occupational therapist in woodworking at a rehab center. "I like to find and share 'secret spots' like the storks outstation in Drenthe," Desiree said. "Biking gives you the opportunity to get in touch with your surroundings. It makes you part of the country you visit, not just a spectator. I ride my bike everywhere, all year round. When I ride my bike, the day becomes mine!"

If You Go

▶ **Getting There:** Most visitors fly into Amsterdam, which is served by most international carriers. Haarlem is just a twenty-minute train ride from Amsterdam.

▶ **Best Time to Visit:** Tulips are in the height of bloom in mid to late April, though weather can be uncertain. Summers are a bit warmer and drier, though the weather is never particularly balmy in the Netherlands.

▶ **Guides/Outfitters:** Several tour operators lead trips to the Netherlands, including Austin-Lehman Adventures (800-575-1540; www.austinlehman.com).

▶ **Level of Difficulty:** The trip above entails six days of riding for an average of 25 miles (40 km) a day. It's rated easy.

▶ **Accommodations:** The Netherlands Board of Tourism and Conventions (+31 70 370 57 05; www.holland.com) lists lodging options throughout the country. Kasteel de Havixhorst (www.dehavixhorst.nl) is a highly recommended property in the province of Drenthe.

DESTINATION

30

NEW YORK CITY

RECOMMENDED BY **Andrew J. Bernstein**

Andrew J. Bernstein's two-wheel connection to New York City goes back a good ways, as he described: "My dad was a cycling enthusiast, and when I was old enough to wear a helmet—about eighteen months—he'd put me in a kid seat on the back of his Motobecane and off we'd go. We'd ride from Brooklyn Heights, where we lived, out to the Verrazano-Narrows Bridge, pausing in Coney Island before pedaling along Sheepshead Bay, and then home. I recall watching the water breaking on the seawall as we rode along the bike path to the Narrows, feeling the breeze and getting to see parts of the city—the industrial and shipping sections; Fort Hamilton, the old military installation at the Verrazano-Narrows; and the amusement parks on Coney Island, all the while sharing the day with our fellow city dwellers. Being a passenger on Dad's bike cultivated my love of Nathan's hot dogs and gave us countless hours to bond. I didn't think of it this way at the time, of course, but those rides presented us both with a slice of New York City life.

"I continued riding—eventually graduating to my own bike—and by the time I got to high school, I wanted to try bike racing. I bought a used road bike and went to Brooklyn's Prospect Park, which was designed by Frederick Law Olmsted, the creator of Central Park. I prefer Prospect to Central Park, as it feels more natural to me. The park is a great resource for cyclists, as it's closed to traffic for most of the day; there's a nice 3-mile loop; and you can always find someone to ride with. From March until September, there are early-morning races there on most weekends, and competing in those events taught me a lot about the nuances of riding—drafting, sprinting, and how to shift. It also exposed me to the greatest aspect of New York riding—its diversity. In New York City, cycling is not the sole province of any one group; everyone from Wall Street types who prize the latest and greatest bikes, to people of much more modest means, are out riding.

DESTINATION

31

There's incredible racial and ethnic diversity among riders—people of all origins and descents. Relative to most places I've ridden—upstate New York, New England, California, Texas, and Colorado among them—this diversity is unusual in a wonderful way. On race mornings, you hear chatter in English, Spanish, and Russian, among other languages. I came to think of it as the 'polyglot peloton'!"

No one would argue that New York is a great city . . . but a great *biking* city? Conventional wisdom might suggest the Big Apple is well-suited for thrill-seeking bike messengers eager to do battle with the endless armadas of taxicabs (13,000 and counting) sweeping down Fifth Avenue. "I would suggest that people avoid riding through Midtown in the middle of the day," Andrew continued, "but there are still plenty of opportunities to ride. There's an extensive network of bike paths in the city, and many bike shops you'll come upon will share a map. Many of those bike paths link different neighborhoods." According to the New York City Transit Bureau, the city now boasts more than 700 miles of bike lanes, with 250 miles added since 2006. In response to growing demand—and in an effort to create a greener Apple—New York has launched a bike-sharing program. In its first phase, the program will consist of 600 stations and 10,000 bikes in Manhattan and Brooklyn.

New York's web of bike paths can help you explore the far reaches of the city. There are also a number of group rides each year, including the Five Boro Bike Tour, Tour de Brooklyn, Tour de Bronx, and the NYC Century Bike Tour, which claims to be the nation's only all-urban 100-mile ride. A favorite route for many riders follows the Hudson River, along the Hudson River Greenway, which stretches from the Staten Island Ferry terminal near the southern end of Manhattan to Inwood Hill Park, at the island's northern tip. "I found my way to the Westside bike path as I got bored riding around Prospect Park," Andrew said. "There are many parks along the way, and in the warmer months, you can stop and rent a kayak and head out on the Hudson. The ride can turn into what I consider to be New York City's most iconic ride. You cross the George Washington Bridge, enjoying views of the city along the way, and then dip briefly into New Jersey. The bridge lets you off at Riverside Park, where there are boat basins and hiking trails and tremendous views of the river. If you're looking to do some miles, you can continue north along the Hudson on Route 9W, on up to Piermont, New York, where there are a number of places to grab a muffin or a drink. There's a good shoulder along the way. Best of all, it's a very social ride; on a pleasant day, you'll see hundreds of cyclists heading to Piermont."

Mornings present a special time of quiet and solitude—relatively speaking—in Gotham. It's a wonderful time to be on your bike, as Andrew described. "My favorite time to ride is in the early morning. This is a time when you *can* ride through Times Square without undue stress, to experience the solitude of cycling simultaneously with the density of New York. Some of my favorite biking moments in New York have been on the Brooklyn Bridge, crossing into Manhattan. The bike path is a wooden boardwalk; you can hear the boards slapping under your wheels. There's an incredible view, as all of Lower Manhattan spreads before you. Though it can be incredibly busy later in the day, there have been times when I'm the only person there in the morning."

ANDREW J. BERNSTEIN is gear editor at *Bicycling Magazine* and a lifelong cyclist. He is an elite-amateur road racer, aspiring cyclocross racer, race promoter, and dedicated bike commuter. As a cycling journalist, Andrew has reported on professional racing, bicycle technology, and culture. He keeps riding because of the opportunities it affords him to explore new places and to meet new people. "No matter where I've been, I've always met incredible people through cycling," he said. Andrew's greatest goal is to help more people to enjoy cycling, and to understand the many benefits that can come when you park your car and ride a bike. He is a graduate of Skidmore College and is currently based in Emmaus, Pennsylvania.

If You Go

▶ **Getting There:** The New York metro region is served by all major airlines.

▶ **Best Time to Visit:** Clement temperatures await from May through October.

▶ **Guides/Outfitters:** Bike and Roll (212-260-0400; www.bikenewyorkcity.com) offers guided rides around the city. Resources for self-guided rides are available at Bike New York (www.bikenewyork.com).

▶ **Level of Difficulty:** Give yourself at least three days to explore New York by bike. Riding is rated easy to moderate.

▶ **Accommodations:** NYC & Company (212-484-1200; www.nycgo.com) lists thousands of accommodations in the metro region.

SOUTH ISLAND

RECOMMENDED BY **Paul Smith**

Peter Jackson's *Lord of the Rings* trilogy showed the world what many Kiwis already knew—that the western portion of the southern island of New Zealand is an area of incomparable natural beauty. The combination of steep mountains, dark green forests, snowcapped peaks, foaming waterfalls, and fingers of blue fjords makes the region one of the most visually stunning, temperate areas in the world. The South Island has long attracted hearty adventurers, most notably trekkers; it's home to two of the world's most beautiful hikes, the Milford Track and Routeburn Track. Anglers also regularly make the pilgrimage to the South Island to fish its clear, uncrowded streams, home to oversized brown and rainbow trout—émigrés from Europe and California. Cyclists will not be disappointed by the riding options—particularly the route that leads from Punakaiki to Queenstown.

"I rode the west coast of the South Island the first time more than twenty years ago," Paul Smith began, "and was struck by two things. First, I was amazed by the incredible diversity of the landscape. Over the course of a week's riding, it's as if you're visiting five different states—California, Alaska, Oregon, Montana, even the big island of Hawaii. You encounter about every ecosystem but desert; though on the final days as we ride through the South Island's Pinot Noir country, you get close! Every day is different, and every day is a treat. The other thing that struck me is that reaching the western edge of the island is like stepping back in time, say, to the 1950s. People in New Zealand (or from elsewhere) move to the west coast for a certain lifestyle—a slower pace and an existence that's a little closer to the land . . . maybe the same reasons that people might move to the Olympic Peninsula or Alaska. There aren't many people in the region—just little coal-mining, gold-mining, or timber towns every 18 or 25 miles (30 or 40 km). The only thing

145

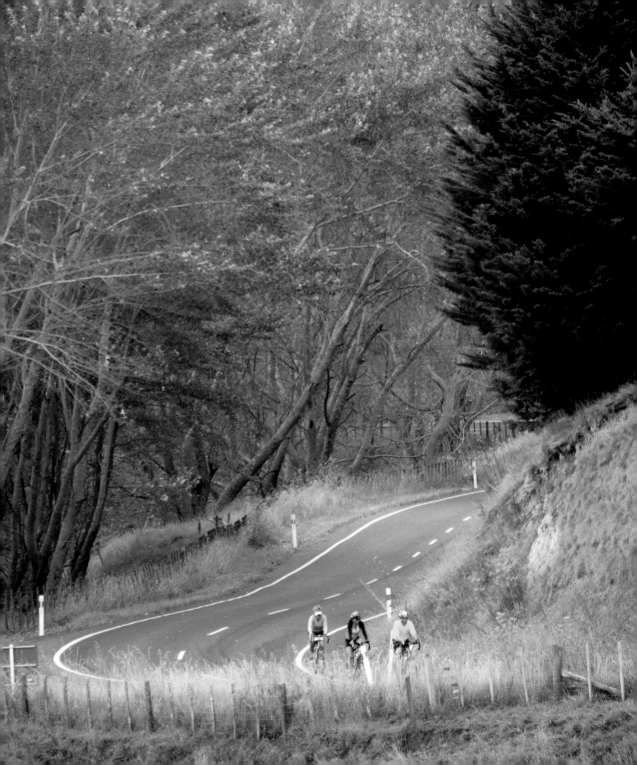

in the middle are dairy farms, scenic reserves, and national parks! Not everyone is cut out for life in Alaska; many Kiwis aren't cut out for life on the west coast. For someone from North America, it may take a while to follow the Kiwi accent . . . and it can take a few more days to sort out that classic west coast sound! Sort of like when you travel down South in the U.S., to, say, Texas or Alabama. But the people are friendly and very curious about us cyclists. They think we're a bit crazy—'You're riding your bike all the way down there? Good on ya!'"

After staging in Christchurch and taking the TranzAlpine train to the island's west side, the ride begins near Punakaiki, at the Pancakes Rocks in Paparoa National Park. "The layered limestone here are unique and resemble—well, pancakes," Paul continued. "On a clear day you can see what lies ahead, Mount Cook and Mount Tasman (New Zealand's two tallest peaks), some 125 miles (200 km) down the coast. Heading south, you experience the Big Sur–like portion of the ride. There are three or four headlands we tackle that are a half-mile to a mile (1 or 2 km) climb each. The road—State Highway 6—hugs the coastline, and the Tasman Sea is crashing below. In places there are sea stacks, like you find along the northern Oregon coast. It's very dramatic, and people generally aren't ready for it. We spend that evening in Hokitika, which has many artists; it's especially noted for its jade carvings and the number of pubs in town! From Hokitika, the road moves inland toward Franz Josef Township—the beginning of the Alaska section of the trip. Farmland gives way to the big, old Kiwi podocarp forest, with rimu, kaihitatea, and other conifers. You feel like you're riding into a national park, and you are—Westland Tai Poutini. As you reach the town at Franz Joseph, you feel the presence of the glacier—it comes right down into the forest close to the back of town. There's a layover day here to explore Franz Josef glacier valley or ride out to the seaside hamlet of Okarito. Between the rain forest, the glaciers, the mountains, and the coast, I've never seen such a variety of terrain within such a short distance."

One of the South Island's more challenging rides awaits as you leave Franz Josef and head south—the Fox Hills. You'll gain 2,100 feet as you pass through lush forest; on clearer days, you'll see Mounts Cook and Tasman just outside of Fox Glacier Township, this time dizzyingly close. The last few hours of this day will be easier on your legs, and your eyes will feast on some of New Zealand's most pristine country en route to Lake Moeraki and the Te Wahipounamu–South Westland National Park, a World Heritage area. "You've left the Alaska-like habitat now, and you're going through one of New

OPPOSITE:
The South Island's west coast has incredible landscape diversity; some sections resemble California, while others, Alaska.

DESTINATION

32

Zealand's most isolated regions," Paul said. "You're surrounded by the forest, and you get little glimpses of the sea and pass by grand lakes and rivers." Many will choose to linger at Lake Moeraki for an extra day, where you can explore spectacular beaches that are home to fur seals and Fiordland crested penguins or delve deeper into the lowland rain forest habitat that's been protected as part of Westland National Park. But the best is yet to come.

"The ride from Haast to Lake Wanaka is one of my favorite rides in the world," Paul added. "I'd put it up against any 90 miles (147 km) in the world for scenery. It starts in the glacial moraine at the mouth of the Haast River. The road follows the river inland as you climb through stands of podocarpus, then into a beautiful beech forest. There's a long stretch of steep climbing that brings you past waterfalls and over rushing streams as the peaks of the soaring Southern Alps rise around you. Finally, you reach the Haast Pass, the South Island's Main Divide (like North America's Continental Divide). On the other side of the pass you drop into the drier country of the Makarora River valley. This area reminds me of Montana, as there are fewer trees, big rocky mountains, and large rivers and lakes. Two of the lakes, Wanaka and Hawea, are reminiscent of Lake Louise in Banff, with its incredible teal waters. Still, there's hardly anyone living here. I'm always left wondering why people don't live here, it's so incredibly majestic. This is the ride that always brings me back to the South Island. I've done it more than fifty times." After a night at picturesque Lake Wanaka (and perhaps an extra day to enjoy some hiking, fly-fishing, or a "flightseeing" tour of nearby Milford Sound), you'll ride through the Otago Pinot Noir region (originally sheep country, now the South Island's Willamette Valley in Paul's opinion) en route to the adventure hub of Queenstown, which might be considered the island's Aspen or Jackson Hole.

"The weather is not always ideal on the west coast," Paul added. "I've had thirteen days of rain in a row, and you can have a cold front come through at any time and foul things up for a bit. But on the back side of the fronts, there's usually four or five days of fine weather. To me, it's all part of the drama of cycling in this very dramatic place."

PAUL SMITH has led more trips than anyone in Backroads' history. Married to another longtime Backroads leader—and now a dad to two sons—Paul has been sharing his passion for China, Bali, New Zealand, and the Pacific Northwest for two decades and looks forward to new discoveries with every visit. A history major and a former minor league

DESTINATION 32

baseball player, Paul is renowned for his attention to detail, witty humor, knowledge of the local haunts, and uncanny ability to discern the needs of each guest.

If You Go

▶ **Getting There:** Visitors generally fly into Christchurch and fly out of Queenstown. Air New Zealand (800-262-1234; www.airnewzealand.com) offers service to both cities.

▶ **Best Time to Visit:** People ride the west coast from late November to mid-March; Paul has found the latter part of the season to provide the most reliable weather.

▶ **Guides/Outfitters:** Many companies lead bicycle trips on the South Island, including Backroads (800-462-2848; www.backroads.com).

▶ **Level of Difficulty:** The route above involves eight days of riding a minimum of 26 to 46 miles (42 to 74 km) a day. It's rated moderate to difficult.

▶ **Accommodations:** Tourism New Zealand (www.newzealand.com) lists lodging options throughout the South Island. Some properties Backroads likes include: in Franz Josef, Te Waonui Forest Retreat (+64 3 357 1919; www.tewaonui.co.nz); in Lake Moeraki, Wilderness Lodge Lake Moeraki (+64 3 750 0881; www.wildernesslodge.co.nz); in Lake Wanaka, Edgewater Resort Hotel (+64 3 443 0011; www.edgewater.co.nz).

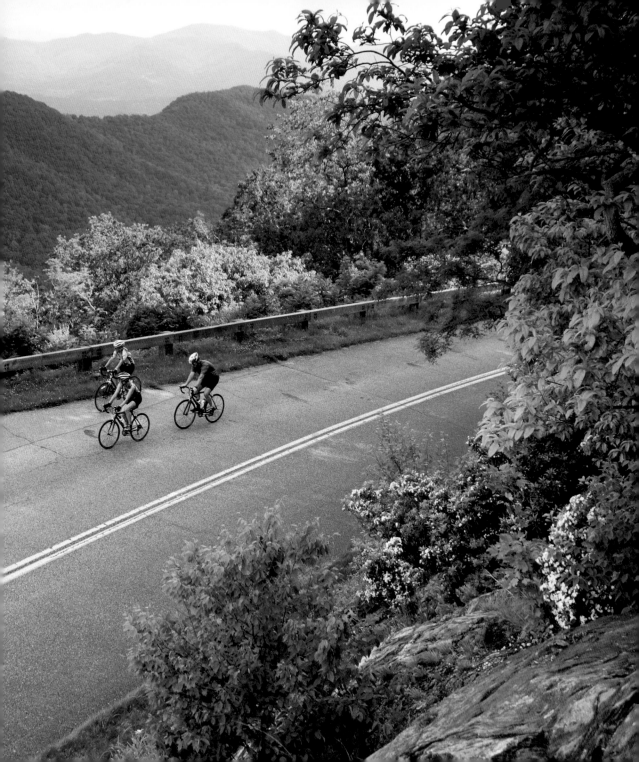

BLUE RIDGE PARKWAY & BEYOND

RECOMMENDED BY **Rebecca Falls**

Stretching 469 miles (755 km) from Shenandoah National Park in the north to Great Smoky Mountains National Park in the south, the Blue Ridge Parkway is one of America's great roads. Ranging in elevation from 600 to 6,000 feet, the Blue Ridge is also one of the east coast's great cycling training grounds, both for professionals seeking to regain their edge and everyday bikers searching for a special challenge. "The Blue Ridge Parkway is like an Appalachian Trail for bikes," according to Rebecca Falls. "There's no commercial activity at all, though if you exit the parkway at the right places, there are colorful towns with all the amenities you need. Cyclists know the road for its climbs—they're long, but not supersteep. As you follow the ridges high up in the mountains, you have tremendous views to the east and west. I've done most of my riding on the southern end of the parkway. Living in western North Carolina, I've gotten to know some of the lesser-known rides in the area. When I got the chance to design a trip for Trek Travel, I wanted to include some of my favorite sections of the Blue Ridge with routes that showcased other aspects of this part of the world." (The blue of the Blue Ridge, incidentally, comes from the haze that's caused by hydrocarbons released into the atmosphere by trees; in the last half century, the haze has increased significantly thanks to man-made pollutants.)

The adventure stages start in Asheville, North Carolina, an eclectic mountain resort town where New Agers, outdoor enthusiasts, and local food advocates all coexist with a patina of southern charm. "It's definitely worth spending a day in Asheville on either end of the ride," Rebecca recommended. "It's a lively scene that you might not expect in southern Appalachia." You'll shuttle to Linville Falls and ride up to your home base for the first half of the trip, the town of Blowing Rock. "There's an interesting story of how the town got its name," Rebecca continued. "The rocky cliffs here were once home to Cherokee and

OPPOSITE:
The Blue Ridge
Parkway has
been described as
an "Appalachian
Trail for bikes."

DESTINATION

33

151

Catawba Indian tribes, who were bitter enemies. The tale goes that a Cherokee boy and a Catawba girl fell in love. One day they were walking near a rocky outcropping. The boy, torn between his loyalty to his tribe and his love of the maiden, jumped from the rock, but the prevailing winds blew him back up into his lover's arms. It's still very windy at Blowing Rock, and the fog can roll in too, even in late spring. It's a true mountain town."

From Blowing Rock, you'll have the option to test your stamina against one of the climbs that has made the region famous among cycling's cognoscenti—Beech Mountain Parkway. The climb from the burg of Banner Elk to Beech Mountain—a 1,400-foot elevation gain over 3.5 miles (5.6 km)—marked the finish for the final stage of a short-lived race called the Tour DuPont—a contest that helped bring a young American rider named Lance Armstrong to prominence. Armstrong had won the Tour DuPont in 1995 and '96 and seemed poised for further achievements when he was diagnosed with testicular cancer. Though given only a 40 percent chance of survival, Armstrong successfully battled the disease and, by early 1998, had returned to serious training—with mixed results. That April, his coach, Chris Carmichael, and Bob Roll, a friend and fellow racer, brought him to the town of Boone for a week of riding in hopes of helping him rekindle his cycling fire. Reaching the top of Beech Mountain one morning during his stay, Armstrong had an epiphany—he was ready to race again. "The ride up that mountain changed everything . . . I was a bike racer again," he wrote in his autobiography. "If I ever have any serious problems again, I know that I will go back to Boone and find an answer."

Whether Beech Mountain presents answers or prompts new questions, you'll experience a more intimate side of the western North Carolina riding experience on day three. "I like to head north and take us off the parkway, as I think it's even more beautiful," Rebecca continued. "On the Blue Ridge, the climbs and descents are gradual in a sweeping sort of way. The roads off the parkway are steeper, with more twists and turns. You're often riding along mountain streams, so you get a denser, more canyon-like feeling than when you're on the parkway above everything. In the spring, the rhododendrons and mountain laurel are blooming, and on the smaller roads, you're right among them. We head toward the community of Idlewild, which has a totally different feeling than Blowing Rock, much more pastoral. From here, it's a shuttle back to Blowing Rock so we have time to do a hike on the Boone Fork Trail in the shadow of Grandfather Mountain. It's nice to have a few hours off the road and to have a chance to enjoy a more backcountry experience."

On day four, you'll leave Blowing Rock and retrace part of your earlier path to Linville Falls, and then on to Lake Lure. "It's a long mileage day, up to 82 miles (132 km), though you lose more elevation than you gain," Rebecca said. "The last stretch takes you through beautiful rolling farmland until you reach Lake Lure, in the Hickory Nut Gorge. The lodge where we stay rests right on the lake, with mountains—including Rumbling Bald Mountain—all around. The Lake Lure region is celebrated for its many outdoor amenities, and after a shorter morning ride on day five, cyclists will have time to take a hike, go fly-fishing or horseback riding, do some rock climbing on the boulders or routes at Rumbling Bald . . . or just relax by the lake."

REBECCA FALLS is a full-time guide and trip design coordinator for Trek Travel. She has worked for Trek Travel since 2004, and enjoys the opportunities that bike guiding has given her to meet amazing people, to travel, and really get to know the areas where she's been fortunate enough to work. These regions range from southern France to the Utah desert. She started working at the Cycle Path, a bike and outdoor shop in her hometown of Tuscaloosa, Alabama. She spent several seasons at the Nantahala Outdoor Center near Bryson City, North Carolina, and currently lives in Asheville, North Carolina, with her husband, Sam, and their cat, Theodore.

If You Go

► **Getting There:** Fly into Asheville, which is served by several airlines, including American (800-433-7300; www.aa.com) and Continental (800-523-3273; www.continental.com).

► **Best Time to Visit:** May through October, though in lower elevations, summer months may be a bit warm and humid.

► **Guides/Outfitters:** Many tour companies lead trips along the Blue Ridge Parkway, including Trek Travel (866-464-8735; www.trektravel.com).

► **Level of Difficulty:** The trip above entails five or six days of biking averaging roughly 40 miles (64 km) a day. It's rated moderate to difficult.

► **Accommodations:** Rebecca recommends the Chetola Resort (828-295-5500; www .chetola.com) in Blowing Rock and the Lodge on Lake Lure (828-625-2789; www.lodge onlakelure.com) in Lake Lure.

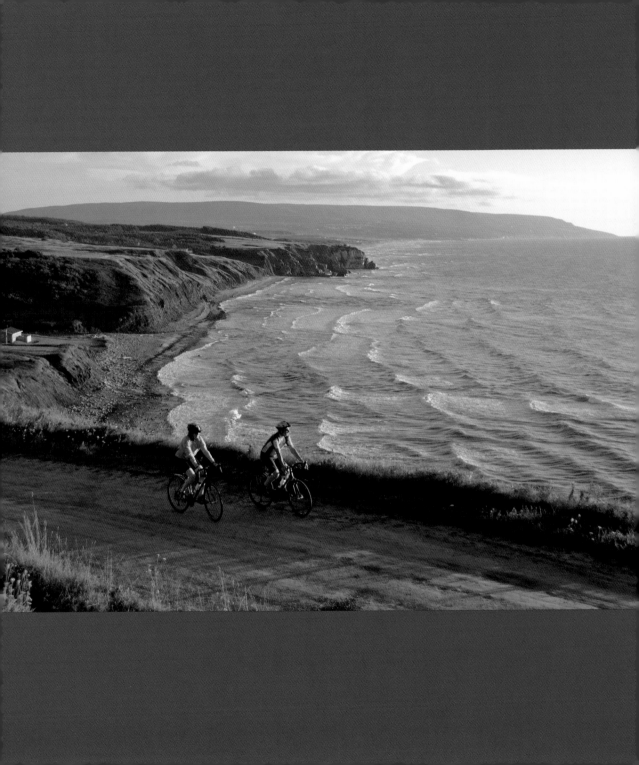

CAPE BRETON

RECOMMENDED BY **Gary Conrod**

Some come to Cape Breton for its rugged coastal mountains. Many come for unparalleled ocean views. Gary Conrod certainly appreciates these facets of Cape Breton, but sees another benefit for cyclists—its human scale. "People still matter here," he began. "There are so few people on the island, you can feel your presence here. On much of the eastern seaboard of North America, people don't have much access to the ocean. There are few places where you can have it all to yourself. Cape Breton is one of those places. Here, you can stand above the ocean, hear the water. It's what people want, even if they don't know it. There's a lack of cars here, no *honk-honk*, and you can ride in peace and quiet. Some ask me, 'What about the trucks on Cabot Trail?' I respond, 'What trucks?' There's no reason for trucks to be there, as there are very few people. The few people who are here take notice of you. You might have people pull over as you're riding along and say, 'Hey, we saw you two days ago in Ingonish, how's it going?' For me, Cape Breton inspires a level of contemplation. You go home changed a bit, more solid than when you arrived."

Cape Breton comprises the northeastern section of the Canadian Maritime province of Nova Scotia. An island unto itself separated from Nova Scotia proper by the narrow Strait of Canso, Cape Breton is bordered by the Atlantic Ocean to the east and the Gulf of St. Lawrence on the west, and is blessed with pine-covered mountains, deep river canyons, and steep cliffs that fall away to the sea; it's regularly recognized as one of the Northern Hemisphere's most beautiful islands. The Cape Breton Highlands encompass the northern section of the island, much of which is given over to 367-square-mile Highlands National Park. Thanks to a cool maritime climate and mountainous terrain, the park hosts a unique blend of Acadian, boreal, and taiga habitats and an incomparable blend of mountain and seascapes. "I have traveled around the globe," Scottish inventor

OPPOSITE:
It's no wonder that the Cabot Trail is considered one of the world's most beautiful roads.

DESTINATION

34

Alexander Graham Bell once wrote. "I have seen the Canadian and American Rockies, the Andes, the Alps, and the Highlands of Scotland, but for simple beauty, Cape Breton outrivals them all!"

If there is one ride that defines Cape Breton and Nova Scotia for cyclists, it's the Cabot Trail. The trail, 185 miles (298 km) in length, loops around the northern tip of Cape Breton and through Cape Breton Highlands National Park. (Construction of the road began in the 1920s as part of the Canadian government's focus on tourism development in the Maritimes; it was completed in its initial form in 1932.) "Everyone who visits wants to do the Cabot Trail," Gary continued. "Many riders will do it in three days. I suggest taking four to six days so you can stop to snap photos, take swims, and explore the many viewpoints and side routes available. Communities are spread out, roughly 31 miles (50 km) apart. If you're going inn to inn, you have to plan ahead to secure accommodations and commit yourself to making the necessary miles. When I do the trail, I like to camp, as it gives you more flexibility."

Many will start the ride near the town of Baddeck in the south and ride up the Atlantic side of the trail. It's not uncommon to see whales as you roll north (fin, pilot, minke, and humpback whales are frequent visitors). At the town of Ingonish, you enter the national park. "You often see animals along the road in the park," Gary said. "Black bear, moose, fox, and coyote. You don't have to look too hard—they come out to you. I once had a moose walk right over me. I'd pulled over and was taking a nap on the side of the road. When I awoke, I was looking up at a moose's belly!" More thrills await as you reach the west side of the park and the Gulf of St. Lawrence. "The ride down French Mountain is exhilarating," Gary added. "The road is very curvy, and there are places where the entire road seems to disappear as you descend—all you see is ocean. You have to slow down if you're not accustomed to the switchbacks. If it's a clear day, you can see all the way to the Magdalen Islands to the northwest."

The Cabot Trail is not your only cycling option on Cape Breton. Gary also recommends the island's west coast from Margaree to Port Hastings, and a ride along Bras d'Or Lake. "There's a fairly new trail there now, and you have the Gulf of St. Lawrence to your right the whole way. The sunsets are spectacular. Some riders will set out to circle Bras d'Or Lake (a part-fresh, part-saltwater body of water in the south center of the island), a ride of 435 miles (700 km). The road is mostly very quiet. A shorter ride that will give you a great sense of this region is from Marble Mountain to Iona, along the top edge of the lake."

Part of the allure of a biking vacation in Nova Scotia is the chance to partake of Cape Breton's thriving Celtic culture. Though it was initially settled by the French in the early 1700s and then ceded to England in 1763, the flavor of the island has been shaped most profoundly by the Scottish immigrants who arrived in the early 1800s. (Oddly enough, geologists believe that Cape Breton may have initially been connected to Scotland millions of years ago!) These Scots, forcibly displaced from the Scottish Highlands, have managed to maintain much of their way of life. While the number of citizens speaking Gaelic is shrinking, the region's culture is being preserved in its music, especially a style of violin playing that's been branded "Cape Breton fiddling," characterized by Natalie MacMaster. The town of Cheicamp is an anomaly, in that it's maintained its old French heritage. "The same French language is used today that was spoken four hundred years ago," Gary added. "They have their own music and food, and both are good. In fact, many of the Scottish musicians like to go there to play, including Ms. MacMaster."

GARY CONROD founded Atlantic Canada Cycling in 1987 to celebrate bicycle touring in Canada's Atlantic Provinces: Nova Scotia, Prince Edward Island, Newfoundland, and New Brunswick. He has cycled almost every road there is in the region and is passionate about sharing the experience. Gary likes to explore places off the tourist route, always the most scenic roads. If there is one less car he will go that way!

If You Go

▶ **Getting There:** Air Canada (888-247-2262; www.aircanada.com) offers daily flights to Halifax, Nova Scotia, from a number of North American cities. From Halifax, it's roughly four hours' drive to Baddeck, the beginning of the Cabot Trail.

▶ **Best Time to Visit:** The roads are generally clear from mid-May through mid-October.

▶ **Guides/Outfitters:** A number of operators lead tours around Cape Breton, including Atlantic Canada Cycling Tours (902-423-2453; www.atlanticcanadacycling.com).

▶ **Level of Difficulty:** The ride above unfolds over eight days, with an average of 44 miles (70 km) a day. It's rated moderate.

▶ **Accommodations:** The Victoria County Department of Tourism website (www.visit victoriacounty.com) lists lodging options in the towns around Cape Breton.

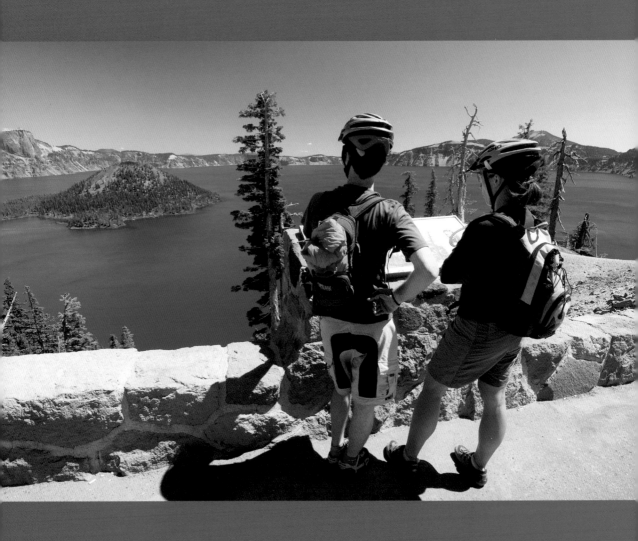

CRATER LAKE

RECOMMENDED BY **Jerry Norquist**

Crater Lake rests at the bottom of a 6-mile-wide, 8,000-foot-tall caldera in the southern Cascade Mountains of Oregon. Shimmering in hues of incredible blue at the bottom of a crater that varies from 500 to nearly 2,000 feet in height, the lake is wonder-of-the-world-inspiring; your first glimpse will leave you speechless! The 33-mile (53-km) loop road that circles the rim resides in the "top ten" rides of many cyclists who've experienced it, and Jerry Norquist is among them. "There are a number of tours you can orchestrate to lead you to Crater Lake," he began. "Some approach from the north—either from the southern Willamette Valley or from the Bend area. I like the idea of starting in the south, beginning and finishing in the town of Ashland. It's such a lovely little town, and there's so much to do when you're not on your bike."

Nestled at the foot of the Siskiyou Mountains 15 miles (24 km) north of the California border, Ashland is a cosmopolitan enclave in the bucolic Applegate Valley. Ashland owes much of its cultural élan to the presence of the Oregon Shakespeare Festival, one of America's oldest professional nonprofit theaters. The theater—which produces eleven plays for nearly 400,000 attendees each year—has drawn a plethora of fine restaurateurs and innkeepers, as well as other performing artists to a town that always had an abundance of outdoor opportunities at its doorstep. After taking in a play or two, you'll head in a northeasterly direction into the Cascades. Some may wish to linger at Lake of the Woods, about 40 miles (64 km) up the road. Surrounded by pine forests, this natural lake has a long history as a summer escape for Oregonians, offering sailing, canoeing, fishing, and hiking. "There are quaint cabins at the lake, and an old-style lodge with all the amenities you need," Jerry continued. "Hard-core riders, however, may choose to continue north on to the village of Fort Klamath."

OPPOSITE:
The 33-mile (53-km) ride around Crater Lake is high on the must-do list for many cyclists.

DESTINATION

35

The ride to Fort Klamath takes you east into a broad, fertile valley that's bifurcated by the Wood River, a spring creek renowned for its trout fishing. With lush, peaceful pastures populated by cattle and big views of the mountains to the east and west, the Fort Klamath region is reminiscent of western Montana. (There's a reconstruction of the town's namesake fort, which was an outpost in the U.S. Army's forays against the Modoc Indians in the early 1870s.) From Fort Klamath, you'll continue roughly 30 miles (48 km) in a northerly direction to the eastern entrance of Crater Lake National Park. Crater Lake is the nation's fifth oldest national park, dedicated in 1902 by Teddy Roosevelt. Once you reach the park border, it's another 7 miles (11 km) to the rim; in this portion of the ride, you climb from 6,000 feet to 7,100 feet; you feel the burn most on the last 3 miles (5 km). But then the lake appears.

There are two stories of how Crater Lake came to be. The Klamath people, one of the Native American tribes that call the region home, tell a legend of two chiefs, Llao of the Below World and Skell of the Above World. They became pitted in a battle, which ended up in the destruction of Llao's home, 12,000-plus-foot-tall Mount Mazama. The mountain's destruction led to the creation of Crater Lake. Geologists believe that an ancient volcano (posthumously named Mount Mazama) erupted. The basin or caldera was formed after the top 5,000 feet of the volcano collapsed. Subsequent lava flows sealed the bottom, allowing the caldera to fill with approximately 4.6 trillion gallons of water from rainfall and snowmelt, creating the ninth deepest lake in the world. Crater Lake sees an average of 44 feet of snow a year; it's the snowmelt that gives the lake its vibrant shades of blue. The Klamath Indians revered the lake and the surrounding area, shielding it from non-native explorers until 1853, when three gold prospectors stumbled upon its waters. (Crater Lake is known as *giiwas* in the Klamath language, which means "spiritual place.") But gold was more on the minds of settlers at the time, and the discovery was soon forgotten. Captain Clarence Dutton, commander of a U.S. Geological Survey party, was the next known Euro-American to visit Crater Lake. From the stern of his survey boat, the *Cleetwood*, Dutton sounded the depths of the astonishingly blue waters with a lead pipe and piano wire. His recording of 1,996 feet was amazingly close to the sonar readings made in 1959 that established the lake's deepest point at 1,932 feet.

After reaching the rim, you'll retire to the regal Crater Lake Lodge, a structure dating to 1915 that's perched above the lake with views of Wizard Island and the surrounding

Cascades peaks. The lobby and dining room, featuring logs with intact branches, certainly complement the Pacific Northwest surroundings. Well-rested and acclimated to the altitude, you'll embark for the famed Rim Drive. "After the elevation you've gained getting to the rim, people often think that the Rim Drive is flat—but it's not," Jerry advised. "In the course of the 33 miles (53 km) you gain almost 4,000 feet, quite challenging for the distance. I always recommend that people ride it clockwise; that way, you get the most views of the lake. At Cloud Cap Overlook, you reach 7,900 feet—the highest point of paved road in Oregon. There are many points along the way worthy of a stop— Merriam Point, Palisades, Pumice Point, Wineglass, and Phantom Ship Overlook. You can stop at the Cleetwood Cove Trail on the north side of the lake and hike down for a boat ride to see the caldera from below. Once you've finished the ride, you can retire to the lodge for another night or continue back toward Ashland. To make it a loop, I like to head west from the park toward the town of Prospect, then Butte Falls and on through the eastern part of the Rogue Valley down to Ashland.

"If there's an iconic moment for me riding Crater Lake, it comes on a clear, crisp day in early June. By this time, much of the Rim Drive is plowed, but there are still 12-foot snowbanks on either side of the road. It's the closest we have in the United States to biking through the great European passes; it's like riding through a snow cave. When I've gone as far as I can go, I turn around and head back to the lodge, put my feet up on the deck overlooking the lake, and enjoy a good Oregon microbrew."

JERRY NORQUIST has been the executive director of Cycle Oregon since 2002. Jerry was involved with the retail and manufacturing side of cycling for more than twenty-five years. He worked for Trek Bicycles and Cycles Peugeot, and was the vice president/general manager of Specialized Bicycles. He is motivated to get more people on bicycles for transportation and recreation.

If You Go

▶ **Getting There:** If you begin in Ashland, fly into Medford, which is served by Horizon Air (800-547-9308; www.horizonair.com) and United Express (800-241-6522; www.united.com), among others.

DESTINATION

35

▶ **Best Time to Visit:** The Rim Road at Crater Lake is usually open enough for bikes by June, and remains accessible until the first heavy snows—generally early November.

▶ **Guides/Outfitters:** Several operators lead trips that include Crater Lake on the itinerary, including Cycling Escapes (714-267-4591; www.cyclingescapes.com) and Bicycle Adventures (800-443-6060; www.bicycleadventures.com).

▶ **Level of Difficulty:** Jerry's trip unfolds over four days of cycling; tours reaching Crater Lake via Bend involve seven days of riding, with an average of 45 miles (72 km) a day. It's rated moderate to difficult.

▶ **Accommodations:** Lodging options along the way include Lake of the Woods Resort (866-201-4194; www.lakeofthewoodsresort.com) and the Aspen Inn (541-381-2321; www .theaspeninn.com). Crater Lake Lodges (888-77-4CRATER; www.craterlakelodges.com) are a must if you can find a room. The Ashland Chamber of Commerce (541-482-3486; www.ashlandchamber.com) lists the many options in Ashland.

CHIEF JOSEPH COUNTRY

RECOMMENDED BY **Jonathan Nicholas**

"We all have certain landscapes or places that speak to us in a special way," Jonathan Nicholas explained. "For some, it might be the Parthenon. For others, Pebble Beach. For me, Chief Joseph Country is one of those signature landscapes. You know when you first set foot here that you're in a place where special things have happened. It's one of the last places where an intact Native American civilization encountered the incursions of an alien culture—it was just 150 years ago. You can still walk in the footprints of the people who came, who saw, who conquered, and drink deep of both the triumph and tragedy of what transpired. As soon as you see the Wallowa Valley, it's immediately apparent why the Nez Perce tribe—and later the settlers—so revere the area. You can understand why, to this day, people fight for the right to live here. All this beauty, all this history, is right there for the taking. You just have to be smart enough to slow down, and the place will speak to you."

For those who think of Oregon in terms of giant Douglas firs and the sea stacks that emerge along its 400-mile coastline, the rugged, wide-open spaces of eastern Oregon come as a surprise. The high desert, punctuated by various mountain ranges (the Alps-like Wallowas, the jagged Elkhorns, the Blues) and Hell's Canyon, North America's deepest gorge, is at once expansive and dramatic. "I first biked there in 1982 while visiting some friends," Jonathan continued, "and I was determined to come back and explore more. I did, and ultimately put together a little tour that I call the Chief Joseph Loop. The circle begins in La Grande, heads south to Baker City, then east to a small town called Halfway, then north to the town of Joseph, and finally west again to La Grande. Accessing this region by bike gives you a sense of the remoteness of the Eagle Cap Wilderness. The climbing—especially on day three—slowly reveals the Wallowa Valley, a remarkable western landscape."

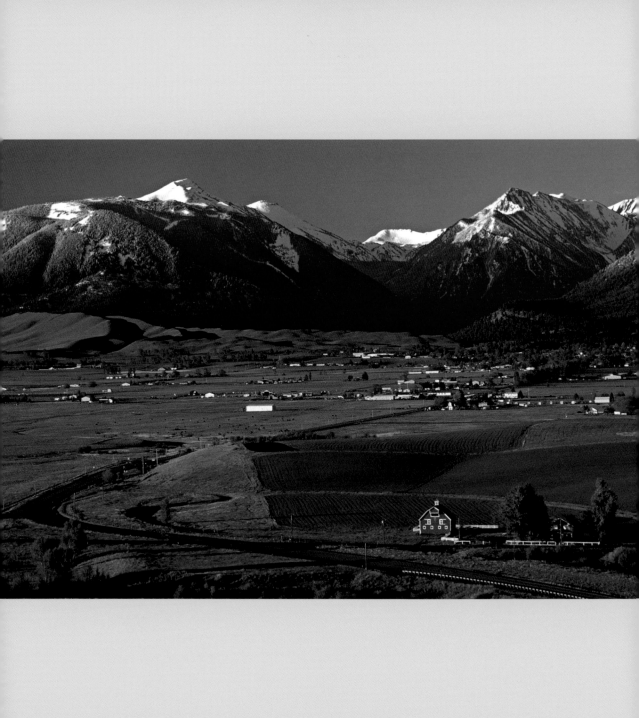

A slightly extended version of Jonathan's route, it's worth noting, is periodically offered by Cycle Oregon, a weeklong biking odyssey that Jonathan helped launch. "In 1988, when I was a columnist for *The Oregonian* newspaper, I resolved to tour rural towns that were being hard hit by changes in the timber industry," he explained. "Clearly, the age of massive timber harvests was over. My plan was to report on how the communities were dealing with this change, and maybe inject a few dollars into those small towns' cafés where too few people were showing up to buy beer and pizza on a Monday night. I mentioned that I was going to do the ride in a column. I thought that perhaps fifty people would join me. One thousand and eight came. And everywhere we went, the story was the same. The smaller the town, the bigger the welcome." It continues today, with Cycle Oregon bringing more than two thousand cyclists to the far corners of the Beaver State each year.

Heading south from La Grande, you get a gradual introduction to the region's remote beauty as you cycle along sylvan Catherine Creek, with the Blue Mountains providing a breathtaking backdrop. Day two begins in Baker City, a turn-of-the-century gold rush town that still boasts much impressive Victorian architecture. On the road out of Baker, you should linger at the Oregon Trail Interpretive Center, where you can literally walk in the ruts of the wagons that carried settlers west to the "promised land" of the Willamette Valley. The route continues north to the town of Halfway, which for a brief time was renamed "Half.com" as an Internet-company marketing stunt. The ride from Halfway to Joseph—day three on Jonathan's itinerary—is particularly awe-inspiring. "The ride is 70 miles (112 km), and has 7,000 feet of climbing," Jonathan described. "You need to be self-reliant, as you can't count on flagging down a passing car if you run out of water—there may not be any! The ride has two significant ascents, but you have the shade of the Wallowa-Whitman National Forest to provide relief as you climb. At the top of the second ascent, you've reached the stunning Hell's Canyon Viewpoint. In my opinion, this is one of the most impressive vistas anywhere. You gaze out across deep, rolling canyon lands, including that remarkable gash carved by the Snake River. The Nez Perce would spend winters down there, following the game—the elk and the deer—as they retreated from the snows of the High Wallowas. Beyond the canyons are the Seven Devils Mountains. To the west you have the snowcapped peaks of the Eagle Cap Wilderness. There are many great vistas on this ride, but the overlook above Hell's Canyon is hard to beat. [According to Nez Perce folklore, Coyote dug Hell's Canyon with a big stick to protect ancestors in

OPPOSITE:
A view over
Wallowa Valley:
one of many
jaw-dropping
vistas in Chief
Joseph Country.

DESTINATION

36

165

Oregon's Blue Mountains from the 'Seven Devils' (mountain range) across the gorge in what is now Idaho.] If you can spare the time, stay an extra night in Halfway. You can ride a variety of loops into the Snake River Canyon, anywhere from 20 (32 km) or 30 miles (48 km) to nearly 100 (160 km).

"From the Hell's Canyon Viewpoint, it's a long, gradual descent into the Wallowa Valley and the town of Joseph (named for Chief Joseph). Joseph has had a renaissance in the past twenty years, earning a national reputation for its bronze foundries and art galleries. But it hasn't lost its spurs-and-saddle soul." Though now, it's true, you can find the great coffee shops and brewpubs that are the new signatures of the Oregon landscape. Cyclists generally stay in town or camp at nearby Wallowa Lake, close to the spot where Chief Joseph is buried. (Resisting forced resettlement from his people's ancestral homeland, Joseph—called Thunder Rolling Down the Mountain in his own language—tried to lead his people to freedom in 1877. After a nearly 1,200-mile journey that military historians still hail as a remarkable example of a fighting retreat, they were apprehended near the Canadian border.) The day four ride takes you along the bucolic floor of the Wallowa Valley—Wallowa translates from the Nez Perce language as the "land of winding waters"—and you'll follow the Wallowa River much of the route. It ends with a spectacular downhill ride back into the college town of La Grande.

"The moment of the ride that always stays with me is the point where you come over the last rise on the Halfway to Joseph stretch. There are a couple of final rollers, then suddenly, the entire Wallowa Valley spreads out below, the wind dancing across the prairie and the sun beginning to set behind the Eagle Caps. It's as if the whole history of the American West is laid out there before you, the place the pioneers called 'The Land at Eden's Gate.'"

DESTINATION 36

JONATHAN NICHOLAS was born and raised in the coal-mining valleys of Wales. He was twelve years old when his grandfather, a coal miner, first took him 1,500 feet underground. "The experience gave me a renewed interest in schoolwork," he said. Jonathan spent four years working on international aid projects in the Himalayas then settled in Oregon, where he spent twenty-six years writing a newspaper column that served as a breakfast staple for the state. In 1988, Jonathan invited readers to join him on a bicycle ride across Oregon. Each September, thousands of cyclists from all over the world now join him on Cycle Oregon. The tour has grown into much more than a charitable effort to bridge the divide between rural and urban. With an endowment of more than $1 million, it serves today as a key change agent forging a role for bicycling in everything from easing traffic congestion and enhancing air quality to fighting childhood obesity and fostering tourism.

If You Go

▶ **Getting There:** Rides around Chief Joseph Country generally begin in La Grande, four hours east of Portland International Airport, which is served by most major carriers.

▶ **Best Time to Visit:** You should find clear roads and clement weather from mid-June through mid-October.

▶ **Guides/Outfitters:** Cycle Oregon (800-292-5367; www.cycleoregon.com) periodically leads trips through Chief Joseph Country.

▶ **Level of Difficulty:** Jonathan's route entails four days of riding, ranging from 60 to 85 miles (97 to 137 kilometers). It's rated moderate to difficult.

▶ **Accommodations:** Travel Oregon (800-547-7842; www.traveloregon.com) lists lodging options along the route and can also provide helpful biking resources.

DESTINATION

36

GREATER PORTLAND

RECOMMENDED BY **Mia Birk**

Touch down in just about any neighborhood in Portland, Oregon, and you'll see cars bearing a bumper sticker that reads KEEP PORTLAND WEIRD. Making bikes an intrinsic part of daily life in the Rose City seems to be part of the "weirdness" equation. "Portland in 2011 is a bit like Paris in the 1920s," Mia Birk began. "We have all these different creative endeavors—sustainable foods, craft beers, ecologically sound architecture, novel land-use strategies, alternative transportation—colliding together, a convergence of activity to shape our world for the better. In the past twenty years, the city has invested significantly in light-rail, in creating walkable neighborhoods, and in setting aside green space. Biking is one piece of the larger puzzle. Portland has a great bikeway network, a well-thought-out infrastructure. I'm on my bike every day, and the network makes it easy to get around. In many cases, I can get places faster on a bike than I would in a car. Even if it takes an extra five minutes, you've gotten your heart rate up, and you feel good doing it. We have a temperate climate, so you can bike all year. Yes, it rains in the winter, but it never rains that hard. Portlanders just put on their rain gear and fenders and go. Our summers are glorious: clear, dry, and seldom more than 80 degrees. And thanks to the urban growth boundaries put in place in the communities around Portland years ago, you can get out to beautiful countryside—mountains or vineyards—very quickly."

Portland rests at the confluence of the Columbia and Willamette Rivers, at the northern end of Oregon's Willamette Valley. For many years Portland lived in the shadow of its flashier neighbors, San Francisco and Seattle, quietly walking its own walk. Recently the city's proximity to the coast and the mountains, its emerging "foodie" culture, and its progressive "green" aura have thrust it into the limelight. (You know you've arrived when a cable program satirizing you appears—enter *Portlandia*!) Many who come to see what some have called the blueprint of cities of the future do so by bike. After all, many bike industry pundits put Portland at the top of the list of American cities for bikeability; Portland has the highest share of bicycle commuters of any large U.S. city (approximately 7 percent—a trend set by iconoclastic mayor Bud Clark in the 1980s, long before it was politically astute) and is the only large city to earn the League of American Bicyclists' platinum status as a bicycle-friendly city.

"When I have guests in town, I like to stay within the city's infrastructure," Mia continued. "One ride I like takes you into the city core. I might begin around Waterfront Park—the acreage of which used to be a parkway—bike south to the Hawthorne Bridge (America's oldest operating vertical lift bridge and one of seven bridges that cross the Willamette), and ride over to the east side of town. From here, I'll head north along the Eastbank Esplanade, which is a favorite for city cyclists, as it's right above the river and offers great views of the downtown area. I'll continue up to the Steel Bridge and then cross back over to downtown. For a longer in-town ride, I may spin out to the Springwater Corridor, a multiuse trail that connects the southeast quadrant of the city to more rural landscapes to the east. Sometimes I'll pull together an informal b-pub tour, or map out an excursion to lots around town where food carts are gathered in pods." A serious tour of Portland's brewpubs can be a daunting adventure—there are more than forty currently operating, more per capita than any city in the world. One must-visit brewpub is Hopworks BikeBar, which is situated on a main bike commuter route in the city's northeast quadrant. The central motif is a fusion of forty custom bike frames (made by local bike builders) over the bar; Hopworks' organic beers have earned many awards. (If you haven't gotten enough of a ride in by the time you reach BikeBar, you can jump on one of a pair of PlugOut stationary bikes and pump some electricity back into the building's grid!) As for food carts, there are some 650, serving everything from Norwegian potato flatbread wraps to Caribbean-style plantains. Many are gathered in groups (pods) of six to ten in parking lots around town.

Between brewpubs, food carts, an abundance of parks and green spaces (including 5,000-acre Forest Park, which is wild enough to sometimes be home to black bears), and a thriving biking culture (be on the lookout for one of PDX's tall-bike enthusiasts; some of these bikes suspend their rider eight or more feet above the ground), it's easy to restrict your riding to the city limits. Yet any number of day trips can bring you in touch with the natural beauty that's so close at hand. One great ride takes you east into the famed

Columbia River Gorge and Multnomah Falls, Oregon's most visited natural site. This ride—roughly 65 miles (105 km) round-trip—first takes you on a bike path along the Columbia River, and then cuts south to the Historic Columbia River Highway. The road is a marvel, both for its visionary engineering and incredible scenery. At the time of its completion in 1922, it was considered "The King of the Roads." On the highway you'll climb into the gorge proper, which stretches 80 miles (128 km) and to depths of as much as 4,000 feet, cutting the only sea-level route through the Cascade Mountain Range. There's a long climb to Crown Point, perched some 900 feet above the river, where you'll enjoy breathtaking views of the gorge east and west. From here, it's a descent of 600 vertical feet past a number of other waterfalls until you reach Multnomah Falls, which cascade 629 feet in two plumes. Many riders also will embark on day (or multiday) tours of Willamette Valley's burgeoning wine country, where Pinot Noirs that are taking the world by storm are being cultivated. Favorite towns on Oregon's wine trail include Dundee and Carlton. Though the industry is growing fast, it's still small enough that you don't feel like the 10,000th person in the door on a given week. (Portland's light rail, The Max, can get you within striking distance of wine country.)

The city has many dramatic biking moments—including the sun reflecting off distant Mount Hood as you ride through the city's west hills or the double rainbows that often appear after a spring shower. One of Mia's favorite moments has more of an everyday flavor, but is no less satisfying. "On winter evenings, I reach the crest of a hill on the east side of town where I live as I bike home from my office," she shared. "Looking down the hill toward the city, I see a nonstop line of blinking lights—all bikes—making their way home. For a proponent of bike commuting, few things could make me happier."

MIA BIRK fell in love with cycling in 1990 while attending graduate school in Washington, DC. Having grown up in suburban Dallas, Texas, she was used to driving everywhere; within a few weeks of getting a bike, she was in the best shape of her life, and a lifelong passion had taken hold. Since then, she has been a dedicated cyclist for recreation, touring, exercise, and daily utilitarian trips. Mia is a principal at Alta Planning & Design, the nation's leading firm specializing in bicycle, pedestrian, and trail planning, design, and implementation. At Alta, she's worked on hundreds of bicycle and pedestrian planning projects around the nation. Mia is also an adjunct professor at Portland State University and founder of the school's Initiative for Bicycle and Pedestrian Innovation.

Before forming Alta, she served as the City of Portland's bicycle program manager. Mia is the author of *Joyride: Pedaling Toward a Healthier Planet*.

If You Go

▶ **Getting There:** Portland is served by most major carriers. Light rail can bring you (and your bike) from the airport to downtown.

▶ **Best Time to Visit:** Portlanders bike year-round, though you'll find the most reliable weather from June through mid-October.

▶ **Guides/Outfitters:** Portland has a plethora of great resources for biking around the city and beyond. These include byCycle (www.bycycle.org), Bike Portland (www.bike portland.org), the Bicycle Transportation Alliance (www.bta4bikes.org), Ride Oregon (www.rideoregonride.com), and Community Exchange Cycle Touring Club (www.exchange cycletours.org). Pedal Bike Tours (503-243-2453; www.pedalbiketours.com) and Portland Bicycle Tours (503-360-6815; www.portlandbicycletours.com) lead trips around the city.

▶ **Level of Difficulty:** Plan at least three days to explore greater Portland, more if you plan to ride the Columbia Gorge or wine country. It's rated easy to moderate.

▶ **Accommodations:** Travel Portland (800-962-3700; www.travelportland.com) lists lodging options in the Rose City.

DESTINATION

37

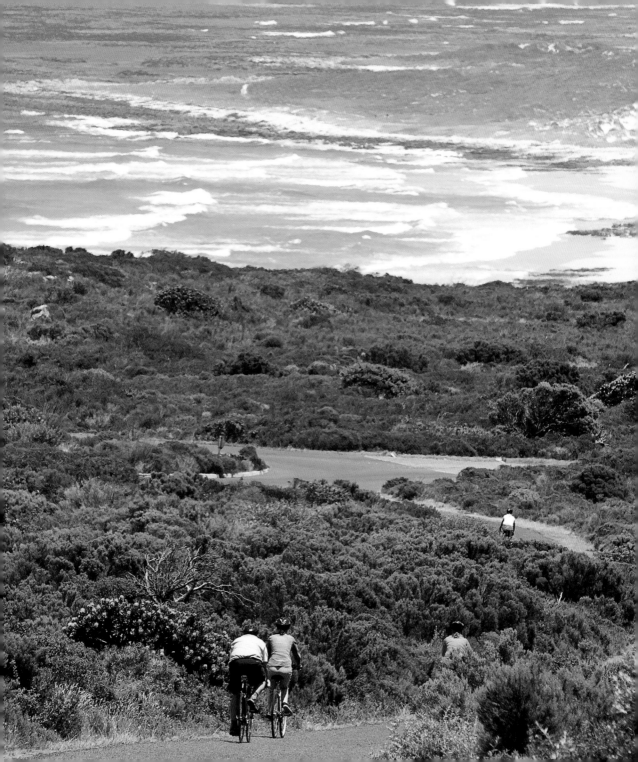

CAPE TOWN

RECOMMENDED BY **Dan Austin**

"Mention Africa and people don't generally think of cycling," Dan Austin began. "They may think of safaris, riding in a jeep across the plains looking at one zebra after another, but not riding a bike. The area around Cape Town will have you reconsidering Africa as a bike destination. The city itself is quite cosmopolitan, a melting pot at the end of the African continent. There's a good biking culture in Cape Town, with many clubs. Thanks to the mild Mediterranean-style climate, there are many professionals training here. Once you get out of Cape Town proper, the roads are very quiet; the average person here can't afford a car. You can ride from hamlet to hamlet along the coast or head in a north-easterly direction to the Winelands region. Or you can stay in town and do day trips— including the famous ride to the Cape of Good Hope."

Cape Town, South Africa's third largest city with a population approaching three million, is situated 20 miles (32 km) from the Cape of Good Hope and is one of the southernmost points on the African continent; the most southerly point is actually at Cape Agulhas, some 90 miles (145 km) southeast. The cape was not settled by Europeans until the 1650s, when the Dutch East India Company established a supply station on Table Bay, in current Cape Town proper. Over the next 250 years, possession of the cape bounced back and forth between the Dutch and the English; the indigenous Khoikhoi people were rapidly displaced in the process. After the Second Boer War (or Anglo-Boer War), Cape Town and South Africa were placed in the Union of South Africa and given commonwealth status; the country gained independence from Great Britain in 1960.

Some people coming to Africa anticipate a third-world experience, but Cape Town is very much a first-world city. Cape Town is framed by Table Mountain, a magnificent natural structure that rises more than 3,500 feet from sea level from a point just a few

OPPOSITE:
The ride to the
Cape of Good
Hope brings you
almost to the end
of the African
continent.

DESTINATION

38

173

miles north of the bay. The main face of the mesa is nearly 2 miles wide. From the top of the mountain (which can be reached on foot or by cable car), you can peer out across the bottom of Africa. The Victoria and Alfred Waterfront—V&A, as Cape Towners call it—is very popular with visitors, somewhat like Fisherman's Wharf in San Francisco. South Africa is celebrated for its beaches, and Cape Town can claim some fine ones, including Clifton, Llandudno, and Boulders Beach; the latter provides a sanctuary for African penguins. As alluded to earlier, Cape Town also has its own wine country roughly an hour outside of the city. One of Dan's "must-do" rides around Cape Town takes you out to the Winelands.

"I like to base myself out of the town of Stellenbosch, which is one of South Africa's oldest settlements [dating back to the late seventeenth century]," Dan continued. "There are fine examples of Cape Dutch architecture here, and wine has been made here for more than three hundred years. You can do several days of riding right from the front door of your inn. Cycling and drinking wine have long gone hand in hand, and there are incredible wineries around Stellenbosch. There are several wine routes. Some of the valleys—particularly Jonkershoek—are quite reminiscent of Napa." There are nearly 150 wine producers in the Stellenbosch region. A few notables include Meerlust Estate, which produces some of South Africa's best Pinotage (a clone created from Pinot Noir and Shiraz grapes); and Thelema, which is best known for its Chardonnay.

The ride that really defines the Cape Town cycling experience, though, takes you out to the Cape of Good Hope Nature Reserve. "The reserve rests on a mountainous peninsula that juts south from Cape Town," Dan explained. "Though it's not more than 20 miles (32 km) from downtown, it's incredibly pristine. Most of the ride to the reserve is downhill. There's lots of wildlife, including Chacma baboons [biologists estimate the presence of eleven troops, totaling 375 animals] and several varieties of ungulates [including Cape Mountain zebra, eland, red hartebeest, and bontebok, which are considered the rarest antelope breed in the world]. You can ride down to Dias Beach, park your bike, and walk 100 yards to the promontory of Cape Point. Here, as you look south, the next land is Antarctica. I remember walking down to the water's edge at the end of my ride out. Here we were, at one of the most southern points on the African continent, and there was such a sense of serenity. No one else was there. There was this profound feeling that we were at the end of the world, and we'd ridden our bikes there. We lingered over a picnic lunch. I felt like I could sit there for days.

"I've cycled next to giraffes and rhinos, and have ridden in many bizarre places. But this was one of the most picturesque spots I've ever visited. Being so close to town yet so far away, it was hard not to contemplate all the trials and tribulations that the people of South Africa have endured."

DAN AUSTIN is the co-founder and director of the award-winning tour company Austin-Lehman Adventures (www.austinlehman.com) which specializes in adult and family multi-sport, hiking, and biking vacations that emphasize history, culture, and nature's charms. In 2009, Austin-Lehman Adventures was named the "Best Tour Operator in the World" by *Travel + Leisure* magazine readers, a recognition the company has repeated for three consecutive years. Dan is also co-founder of the nonprofit Wheels of Change (www .wocinternational.org), which was honored with the *Travel + Leisure* Global Vision Award for 2011. Wheels of Change assists in the collection of used bicycles, parts, and tools that are then shipped to rural communities in Africa to help alleviate poverty, assist in mobility, improve education and health care, and provide jobs and commerce. Dan lives in Billings with his wife, Carol, his daughter, Kasey, and his son, Andy.

If You Go

▶ **Getting There:** Cape Town is served by most major international carriers; most flights from the United States connect via London.

▶ **Best Time to Visit:** November to February (the austral summer) is the most popular time to visit Cape Town.

▶ **Guides/Outfitters:** Austin-Lehman Adventures (800-575-1540; www.austinlehman .com) can customize a bike tour around greater Cape Town.

▶ **Level of Difficulty:** Plan several days to bike around Cape Town, and several more days if you to ride the Stellenbosch region. It's rated moderate.

▶ **Accommodations:** Cape Town Routes Unlimited (+27 21 426 5639; www.tourism capetown.co.za) lists lodging in Cape Town and the Stellenbosch region.

DESTINATION

38

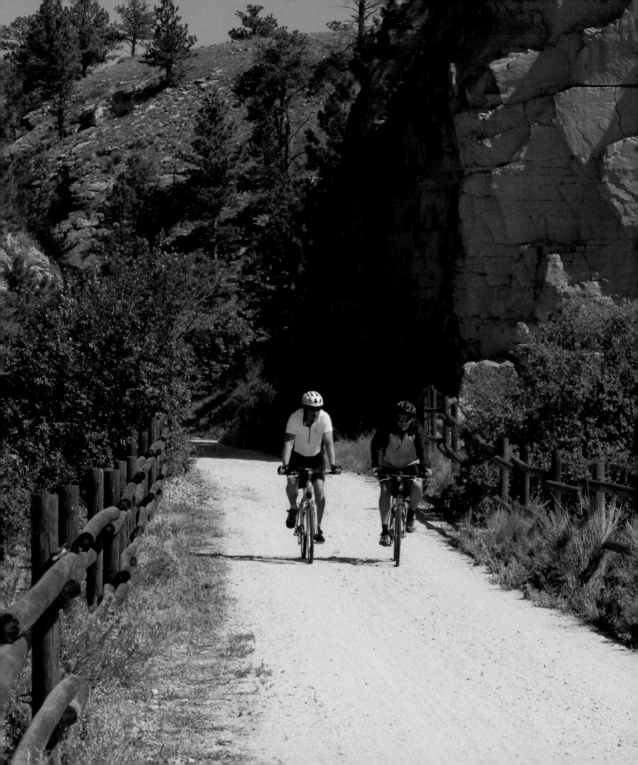

BLACK HILLS

RECOMMENDED BY **Art Brown**

The Black Hills rise abruptly—and some would say, mysteriously—from the plains of South Dakota and eastern Wyoming, an otherworldly alpine island against the endless flatness of the prairie. Summer vacation road-trippers heading for Yellowstone and motorcyclists riding toward the annual rally in Sturgis may pass through, finding the region a welcome respite from the seemingly limitless plains to the east. While they are not a traditional destination for cyclists, more and more self-powered two-wheelers are discovering the Black Hills thanks to the 110-mile (177 km) Mickelson Trail, South Dakota's first rails-to-trails project.

OPPOSITE:
The 110-mile
(177-km)
Mickelson Trail
takes cyclists
through the heart
of the Black Hills.

"Whichever way you're approaching the Black Hills, they jump from the land," Art Brown began. "I've never seen anything like them. I've done trips in Montana and the Canadian Rockies, and when you ride through a mountain pass there, you're seldom above 6,500 feet. There are a number of spots on the Mickelson Trail where you top 6,000 feet, though you couldn't call these sections a pass. The general elevation is simply very high. [The highest point in the Blacks is Harney Peak, which reaches 7,244 feet.] The riding here is visually pleasing, with large forests of ponderosa pine and formidable rock formations. But there's also an Old West feel. Visiting the old saloons or riding through a former railroad tunnel, it's not hard to imagine the Black Hills' rough-and-ready frontier past."

The Black Hills region encompasses 4,500 square miles in western South Dakota, bordered by Interstate 90 to the north and the town of Edgemont in the south. (The name derives not from the shade of the rock, but from the dark color the region's pines presented from a distance.) Once the domain of the Crow, Cheyenne, and Kiowa tribes, the Black Hills were under the control of the Lakota Sioux when whites began exploring the area. The region is sacred to the Lakota, and the United States signed a treaty prohibiting

177

white settlement there in 1868. But when gold was discovered, that agreement was ignored. Prospectors (and the requisite merchants to serve them) descended upon the Black Hills, leading to a series of conflicts, including the Battle of the Little Bighorn to the northeast in Montana. The Lakota were ultimately displaced, and claims were staked throughout the region. By the early 1900s, most of the mines had played out, though some of the boom-time communities—Lead and Deadwood among them—managed to endure. Deadwood will be your first stop after leaving Rapid City. Though its casinos have given the town a slicker veneer than it had in its previous heyday, a little poking around will expose its history. "You can take a tour of the Homestead or Broken Boot gold mines," Art continued, "or visit Boot Hill, where a number of infamous folks are buried, including Calamity Jane and Wild Bill Hickok. You can also stop in for a sarsaparilla or beer at No. 10 Saloon, where Hickok met his end at the hand of Jack McCall. If you have an extra day, you can catch a reenactment of the McCall trial in town."

From Deadwood, you'll join the Mickelson Trail, which showcases a smorgasbord of Black Hills ecosystems, from thick evergreen forests to rocky canyons and prairie-scapes. In its original incarnation, the trail was part of a line built by the Chicago, Burlington, and Quincy Railroad to serve the mines; tracks were initially laid in 1890. Plans for the rails-to-trails project first materialized in 1983, and were championed by Governor George S. Mickelson in his 1986 campaign. The project was green-lighted, but the governor died in a plane crash before the trail was completed in 1998; it bears his name today to commemorate his support. The Mickelson Trail passes through railway tunnels, hugs steep granite walls, and crosses many creeks; overall, there are more than one hundred trestles, some tall enough to give you sweeping views of the surrounding terrain. The trail's maximum elevation is 6,100 feet; riding north to south will help you take advantage of a downward grade. "The quality of the trail from a riding standpoint is superb," Art said, "with a wide, hard-packed surface that you can easily handle with a touring bike. Because it is a former railroad, no grades are greater than 4 percent; I'd say the average is 3 percent, in many places, hardly noticeable, though there are just enough climbs to make it challenging. There are beautiful facilities at each of the trailheads along the way, log cabin–style shelters and pumps to provide fresh well water. As you go south, views open up more as you leave the taller mountains and enter more rolling terrain. The juxtaposition of the ponderosa pine and rocky canyon lands in the north with the prairie in the south is very pleasing." You'll have ample wildlife-viewing opportunities along the trail as bighorn sheep, elk, pronghorn antelope, mountain goats, and mule deer all call the Black Hills home; even mountains lions are occasionally spotted.

"Between Hill City and Hot Springs, our second day on the trail, we pass very close to the Crazy Horse Memorial," Art added. "It's an enormous structure; when it's done, it will be much bigger than Mount Rushmore." The sculpture of Crazy Horse is indeed a monumental work in progress. Polish-American sculptor Korczak Ziolkowski began work in the Black Hills in 1948. He passed away in 1982, and his family carries on the project. In its final form, the memorial will be 563 feet high by 641 feet long, the largest sculpture in the world.

From the southern reaches of the Mickelson Trail, you'll move north, passing first through Wind Cave National Park and then on to Custer State Park. Here, you'll ride along the Wildlife Loop Road, where you have a very good chance to come face-to-face with some of the park's 1,300 bison, which roam freely. "When you're sitting there on a bike and one of these huge animals [bison can weigh a ton] crosses in front of you, you don't have the sense of protection you do when you're in a car," Art said. "It's open range for these guys, and when you come upon them, it's up close and personal." As you continue north toward Hill City, there's an opportunity to see South Dakota's *other* large rock sculpture. "Mount Rushmore is about 2.5 miles (4 km) off the road, near Keystone," Art continued. "The last time I did the ride, none of my fellow riders opted to visit—the weather was too rough. The good news is that Rushmore is close enough to Rapid City that people generally have time to rent a car and drive back to see the four presidents before they fly home."

ART BROWN has served with the Royal Canadian Air Force for more than thirty years. He took up cycling while on exchange with the U.S. Air Force near Sacramento in 1989 and has been a member of Adventure Cycling Association (ACA) since the early '90s. Art eventually took ACA's Leadership Training Course, and has been leading ACA tours in the United States both on and off-road. These trips include Cycle Montana, the Southern Tier, Waterton-Glacier, New Englander Loop, and Great Divide Alpine. He has also ridden in southern France, the Netherlands, Belgium, and Germany. Upon retirement, Art plans to bike from Cairo to Cape Town on the "Tour d'Afrique."

If You Go

▶ **Getting There:** The Black Hills region is most easily reached via Rapid City, South Dakota, which is served by several airlines, including American (800-433-7300; www .aa.com), Delta (800-221-1212; www.delta.com), and United (800-864-8331; www.united .com).

▶ **Best Time to Visit:** You should find clear roads in the Black Hills from June through September. Shoulder months are preferred, as July and August see lots of road traffic. And beware of the Sturgis Motorcycle Rally in August—all rooms will be booked for hundreds of miles!

▶ **Guides/Outfitters:** Several organizations lead trips around the Black Hills, including Adventure Cycling Association (800-755-2453; www.adventurecycling.org).

▶ **Level of Difficulty:** This trip entails six days of riding, with an average of 39 miles (63 kilometers) per day. It's rated moderate.

▶ **Accommodations:** The Mickelson Trail Affiliates website (www.mickelsontrail affiliates.com) lists lodging options along the trail.

DESTINATION

39

LA RIOJA

RECOMMENDED BY **Andy Levine**

"Many Americans visit Spain," Andy Levine led off, "but they tend to spend most, if not all, their time in the cities—Madrid, Barcelona, and Seville. Few visitors get out to the countryside. Here, you see a much different aspect of Spanish life than you encounter in the urban areas. For me, the Rioja region captures the essence of rural Spain. Very few tourists get up to this area. You might pass through a little town of two hundred souls, and come upon a woman beating her rug out the window or hanging her laundry out to dry. The look on her face says 'What are these people on bikes doing here?' Yet the people in these villages are very welcoming. The Rioja also happens to be a place where some great wines—often at a great value—are being produced."

The autonomous community of La Rioja is situated in the north of Spain, roughly 150 miles (240 km) above Madrid. Named for the River Ojai, which flows through the area, the region was once a cultural crossroads. It was here that pilgrims from the north on the Camino de Santiago de Compostelo (Way of St. James)—Celts, Goths, Franks, and Saxons—mingled with Iberians, Romans, and Arabs coming from the Mediterranean, via the Ebro River. The mixing of influences helped shape the region's identity and also forged its wine-growing reputation. Wine has been made in the area for more than three thousand years, with the first vines cultivated by Phoenicians. The importance of wine to the region is underscored by a decree from the mayor of Logroño in 1635, banning carriages from passing along the road next to cellars, "for fear that the vibration from these vehicles might affect the juice and the ageing [sic] of our precious wines." Rioja's vineyards are best known for reds pressed from the Tempranillo grape.

Andy's tour of La Rioja was designed for leisurely riders, people who, in his words, "want to chill out and get into the local culture. It focuses on great cycling roads that bring

181

people to great wines. Cycling is an important sport in Spain, and care is taken to make the roads the best they can be. It's not an overly difficult tour—about 25 miles (40 km) a day—though there are enough hills to work off your meals. There's a nice variety of landscapes—from rolling vineyard lands to drier habitats that would look at home in the American Southwest. I can remember days when I didn't see any cars on the road at all. Pretty countryside, good roads, and real people—for me, that makes good cycling."

After flying into Madrid, riders will generally shuttle to the village of Ábalos, home for the next few nights. The first day of riding takes you along the banks of the Ebro, with a midday break at Bodegas Arabarte. "One thing I've noticed in Spain is that many vineyards seem to invest almost as heavily in their architecture as in their vines," Andy continued. "In France, many of the wineries—even some of the very fine ones—are in these older, somewhat run-down structures. In La Rioja, you'll be riding through this old rustic town and then come upon a winery with wild modern architecture. That's the case at Arabarte." With a taste or two of Arabarte's reds, you'll enjoy a traditional Rioja lunch. This will often include three or four courses: a choice of soup or hors d'oeuvres (called *entremeses*), followed by an egg or fish dish, then a meat course (often lamb) with vegetables, and then a dessert of pastry, custard, or assorted fruit. The day ends with a visit to the medieval walled city of Laguardia, known for its tapas bistros.

The following day's ride takes you to the fortress town of Lerma. En route, you'll cycle through Briones, home of Museo Dinastía Vivanco, a wine museum that features more than three thousand corkscrews, among other exhibits. Passing over the route of the Way of St. James, you'll ride by the monastery of San Millán de la Cogolla, regarded as the birthplace of the Spanish (Castilian) and Basque languages. Your home that night is Parador de Lerma, once a palace that was constructed for King Philip III in the early seventeenth century. Aranda de Duero is your next stop, via the Ribera del Duero wine region, home to two of La Rioja's most celebrated vintages, Tinto Pesquera and Vega Sicilia, both Tempranillos. Dinner will be the culinary focus this day, and as it's generally not served until 9:30, you'll have worked up an appetite. Like the sit-down lunch, the evening meal is generally a four-course affair—soup, fish, then a meat course followed by dessert. You'll have a chance to sample paella, one of Spain's staple dishes. It's rice seasoned with saffron, usually topped with shellfish, chicken, sausage, and peppers.

"My fondest memories of riding in La Rioja involve coming into the little towns in the later afternoon or early evening and watching life unfold," Andy reminisced. "The people don't have much money, but they're very hospitable and festive. In fact, there seems to be a festival going on every night, with vendors making sausages and other tapas, and other vendors selling jug wine. In Pedraza, a hill town dating back to the Renaissance, there's a stone courtyard where everyone gathers to drink wine and be merry. Sometimes there's a bullfight scheduled. People will be gathered together, and all of a sudden a bull will come running through the streets. Soon everyone else will be running along with the bull."

ANDY LEVINE is president and founder of DuVine Adventures, which has been delivering award-winning cycling vacations since 1996. Andy, a true bon vivant with a real passion for adventure, headed to France to hit the open road with his bike and a lust for the good life the day after graduating from the University of Denver in 1992. After leading bike trips in France, Switzerland, and Italy, Andy decided that he could create his own high-quality bike trip without boundaries: a fun combination of biking, drinking, eating, sleeping . . . and of course a little sweat. The first trip booked just two people from Bloomfield Hills, Michigan, whom he led through Burgundy, France. After that the phones never stopped ringing.

If You Go

▶ **Getting There:** Trips for the Rioja region begin and end in Madrid.

▶ **Best Time to Visit:** Riders will find the best weather from mid-April through mid-June and again in September through mid-November.

▶ **Guides/Outfitters:** A number of companies lead trips through the Rioja region, including DuVine Adventures Bicycle Tours (888-396-5383; www.duvine.com).

▶ **Level of Difficulty:** The itinerary above involves five days of riding with an average of 25 miles (40 km) a day. It's rated moderate.

▶ **Accommodations:** DuVine uses the following hotels on its rides: in Ábalos, Hotel Villa de Ábalos (+34 941 334 302; www.hotelvilladeabalos.com); in Lerma, Parador de Lerma (+34 902 54 79 79; www.parador.es/en/parador-de-lerma); in Aranda de Duero, Hotel Torremilanos (+34 947 51 28 52; www.torremilanos.com); in Pedraza, Hospederia de Santo Domingo (+34 921 509 971; www. hospederiadesantodomingo.com).

DESTINATION

40

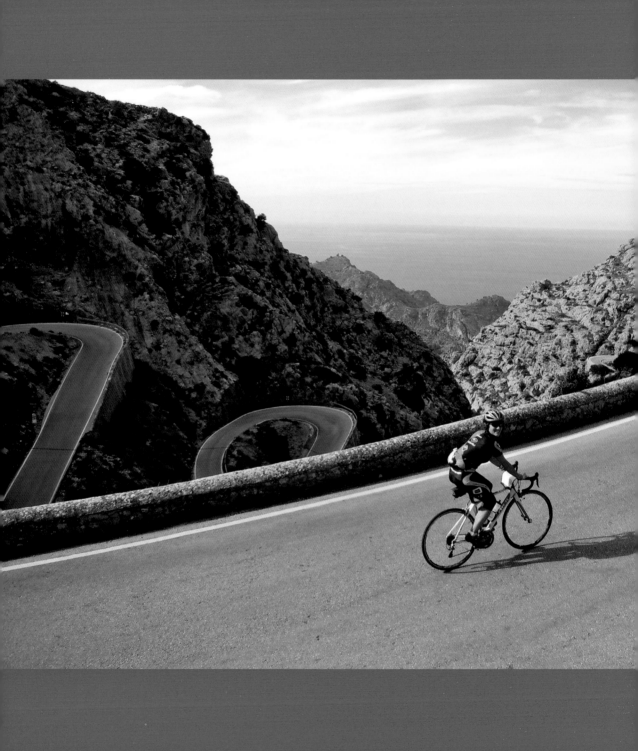

MAJORCA

RECOMMENDED BY **Daniella Soeder**

"After a recent tour of Majorca," Daniella Soeder began, "one of my guests said, 'If Disney was to invent a road bike ride, this would be it!' There's something to this thought. We have many switchbacking roads that twist up and down the mountain passes and along cliffs that hang over the Mediterranean. Add to this a perfect climate, very light traffic, and a unique culture, and you have all the elements of a premier cycling destination."

Majorca is situated some 120 miles (193 km) southeast of Barcelona and is the largest island under Spanish administration. Throughout recorded history, Majorca has been under the sway of the Romans, the Byzantines, the Moors, and now, the Spanish. Residents speak a dialect of Catalan, *Mallorquí*, though Spanish is also to be heard. "People here see themselves as Majorcan first, Spanish second," Daniella continued. "Though many people think of Majorca for its beaches, we have a thriving agricultural area in the center of the island—wonderful fresh fruit and vegetables, as well as lamb and goat. We're especially known for our almonds, figs, and olives. Some of the olive trees here are one thousand years old. The age of the trees gives our olive oil a great complexity." Professional and serious amateur riders in Europe know Majorca as a training destination—both for its climate and its climbs. "On a tour this fall," Daniella added, "we saw both the current world champion (Englishman Mark Cavendish) and the Tour de France winner (Australian Cadel Evans) on their bikes."

Daniella's favorite tour focuses on the northern half of the island, crisscrossing the Sierra Tramuntana. After a night in Valldemossa, one of Majorca's most beautiful mountain villages, you'll embark on the first of several epic rides. "This day, you'll climb through five colls (or passes), each gaining roughly 1,000 feet in elevation," Daniella explained. "There's not a mile of straight road on the route as you twist and turn through olive

OPPOSITE:
Majorca's road
builders seem to
have had serious
cyclists in mind
when they set
to work.

groves and little mountain towns. The roads are very narrow, half the size of a normal one. The speed limit is very low for the few cars that drive them; bikes rule here! The first half of this ride is in the center of the mountains; the second takes you between the Mediterranean and the mountains, with steep drop-offs to the sea. Along the sea, we'll come upon the stone watchtowers that were built in the sixteenth century to monitor the activities of pirates who frequently marauded Majorca. If pirates were spotted, lights would be lit in one tower, signaling other towers along the coast to fire up their beacons. In ninety minutes, the whole island could be alerted. You can tour the towers; from the platform, you look straight down into the sea. The day ends in the town of Deià in the famous La Residencia hotel, high above the Mediterranean."

Your third day of riding takes you over two well-known passes, Coll de Soller and Coll de Horno. "Coll de Soller has thirty-one switchbacks—basically one every 200 yards (183 m)," Daniella continued. "It's equally fun to climb as it is to come down. The ascent to Coll de Horno is in the shadow of Majorca's tallest mountain, Puig Mayor, which stands 4,800 feet. You pass wild rock formations in the limestone, crafted from eons of erosion, as well as narrow slot canyons. The day ends with a fast descent to Monnàber, where we stay at a finca that's a working olive oil farm." The following day will take you farther into Majorca's interior, and will include a stopover in the market town of Sineu, where you can buy anything from a donkey to a silver candelabra. Most of this day is on flatter roads, but toward the end of the day you'll climb to the monastery of Santuari de Sant Salvador, which dates back to 1342. Now converted into an inn, Santuari de Sant Salvador sits at 1,650 feet and has commanding 360-degree views across the island to the Mediterranean. "There was a boy named Guillermo Timoner Obrador who grew up in the village at the bottom of the hill where Sant Salvador sits before World War II," Daniella recalled. "He started riding his bike up the switchback roads to the monastery. Apparently this was good training, because when he grew up, Guillermo went on to become Spain's first cycling world champion and the dominant track rider for a decade. His six rainbow jerseys hang in the monastery. He is revered like a saint!" At Sant Salvador, you stay in a converted monk's cell—a great place to reflect on the day's ride.

After a recovery day that takes you to the walled city of Pollenca, two very memorable rides await. The first takes you to Cap de Formentor, a peninsula jutting to the north. "We ride out to the tip, where there's a lighthouse," Daniella described. "In places, the road hugs a cliff, with the Mediterranean far below. In others, the peninsula is so narrow that you can take in the sea on both sides. It has to be one of the world's most scenic rides! On the way back, I like to ride down to the little fishing village of Cala Sant Vicenç. There's a small seafood bar tucked in among the rocks; they grill up whatever the fishermen have brought in, sometimes fresh tuna." The next day's ride takes you across the northern Sierra Tramuntana, via Coll de Sa Bataia. "The ride starts gently in the foothills, sliding past olive groves and almond trees," Daniella continued. "Then the climb begins. It's not steep—about a 5 percent grade—but it's long, at 5 miles (8 km). At the top, you have the option of returning to Pollenca via the monastery at Lluc, or riding up and down Sa Calobra, the pride of Majorcan road builders. From the top, you wonder how it was possible to construct this road, which clings to the mountain and switches back and twists to the bottom of a steep canyon. The ride back up is a road cyclist's dream, one of the world's great climbs. Many professionals (including Lance Armstrong) have ridden this as part of their spring training. They might take twenty-two minutes to ride up Sa Calobra; if you can do it in forty-five, you're doing well."

DANIELLA SOEDER grew up in Colombia and New York before arriving in Majorca as a teenager. She has worked as a guide on the island for many years, helping to design and lead cycling, hiking, climbing, and kayaking adventures as well as culture tours.

If You Go

▶ **Getting There:** A number of airlines serve Palma de Mallorca, including Air Berlin (866-266-5588; www.airberlin.com) and Ryanair (+44 871 246 0002; www.ryanair.com).

▶ **Best Time to Visit:** You'll find the driest weather June through September.

▶ **Guides/Outfitters:** A number of bicycle tour companies lead trips to Majorca, including Rocky Mountain Cycle Tours (800-661-2453; www. rockymountaincycle.com).

▶ **Level of Difficulty:** The tour above includes seven days of riding, with an average of at least 40 miles (62 km) a day. It's rated moderate to difficult.

▶ **Accommodations:** Rocky Mountain Cycle Tours likes the following properties: in Deià, La Residencia (+34 971 63 9011; www.hotel-laresidencia.com); in Monnàber, Hotel Monnàber Vell (+34 971 51 61 31; www.monnabervell.com); in Sant Salvador, Petit Hotel Hostatgería Sant Salvador (+34 971 51 52 60; www.santsalvadorhotel.com).

DESTINATION

41

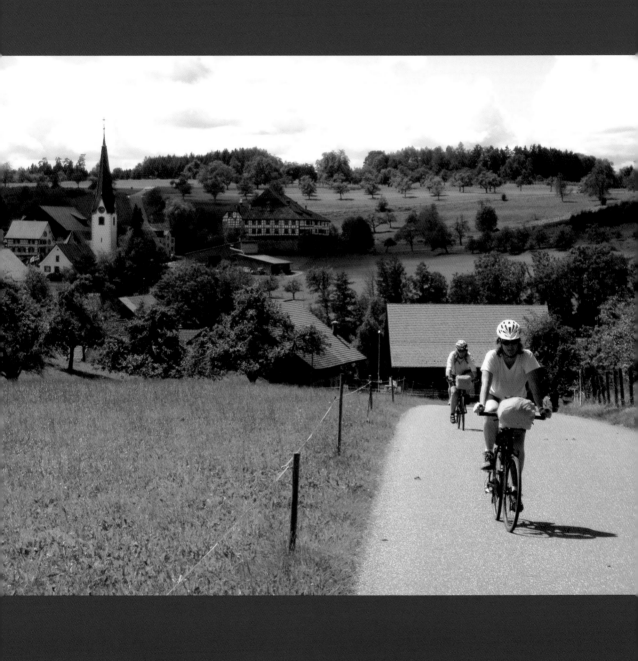

CROSS-COUNTRY TRAVERSE

RECOMMENDED BY **John Klemme**

As exemplified by its watches and banking system, Switzerland is celebrated for an incomparable level of tidiness and efficiency. This passion for orderly precision extends to its cycling system, which helps to make this small landlocked nation (bordered by Germany to the north, France to the west, Italy to the south, and Austria and Liechtenstein to the east) a joy to ride in. "The Swiss have established nine national bike routes and more than fifty regional routes," John Klemme began. "The national routes crisscross the various regions and cantons. There's a committee that goes out and plans the routes, based on traffic density and scenic qualities. Once a route has been established, there's an infrastructure team that develops the bike paths, if necessary, and rest stations with shade and running water. In addition to being well kept, the routes have excellent signage negating 80 percent of any navigational problems visiting riders might encounter. From what I've been told, Switzerland may have one of the world's best-subsidized cycling infrastructures. Biking is certainly respected. I recall being on a train once, and a passenger complained about our bikes blocking the door. I said in German, 'You have something against cyclists?' His face went white; it's not politically correct to be anti-bicycle. Everyone has a bike in their garage; a serious cyclist may have two or three."

Over the years, John has assembled a number of cross-country itineraries in his adopted home. "When I was twelve, my dad took me on RAGBRAI® (see page 99), and it was my first multiday bicycle ride," John recalled. "When I started Bike Switzerland, I wanted to do something that would take people across the country, as RAGBRAI takes people across Iowa." One of his favorite routes travels from Lake Geneva in the west to Lake Constance in the northeast. "Riding RAGBRAI, we used to dunk our tires in the Missouri River on the western edge of the state as we began, and in the Mississippi on the eastern

OPPOSITE:
Switzerland offers cyclists a carefully conceived bike route system that encompasses nine national routes.

DESTINATION

42

edge at the completion. On this ride, we do the same with the two lakes. The ride combines sections of National Routes 1 and 9: the Rhone and the Lakes Routes. We call it our 'Challenge Tour,' and as the name implies, it's best-suited for those seeking a challenge. There's some climbing on most days, but nothing too scary. When people think of biking in Switzerland, they're often intimidated by all the mountains. The truth is there are many doable itineraries. If you ride 800 to 1,000 miles a year, the ride is accessible."

Leaving from Geneva, you'll pass along the northern shores of Lake Geneva (Lac Léman for the Swiss) toward the beautifully terraced vineyards of the Lavaux region. "If it's a Saturday, there are usually festivals, markets, and sporting events in progress in the little towns you pass through," John continued. "It's a great chance to get a sense of Swiss culture. The first 50 miles (80 km) are fairly flat, but you gain about 1,000 feet as you climb to the small town of Chexbres. En route, I like to stop in Lavaux, where you can sample a chilled white wine from the surrounding vineyards at the Maison du Vigneron. I recommend staying in Chexbres; the view of the lake surrounded by snowcapped mountains sets the mood for the rest of the ride." The following day, you'll proceed along Route 9 to Gstaad, the ski resort/playground of the rich and famous tucked in the shadow of the Bernese Alps. You may wish to stop for a chocolate treat at a local café as you depart Gstaad, but you'll surely want to linger in the medieval village of Gruyères, known for its signature cheese, as well as its castle, which dates back to the thirteenth century. (Tours are available at the cheese factory.)

The following day takes you through several beautiful Swiss valleys before you arrive at Interlaken. "We follow streams through pastures on car-free gravel paths. There's plenty of time to stop and pat the noses of the cows working hard to make that delicious cheese! Few visitors get to experience these valleys as cyclists do. Most only see the valley from the trains that run from Montreux to Interlaken." Once you arrive in Interlaken, John recommends leaving your bike at the train station and taking the cogwheel train up to Wengen for a day or two of hiking. "It's good to mix things up a bit," John advised. Wengen is one of Switzerland's more serene alpine villages, and is off-limits to cars. The following day, it is back on the trail along Lake Brienz. "This route is called the Lakes Route because we pass by so many: Lake Thun, Lake Lucerne, Lake Zug, Lake Zurich, Lake Constance, Lake Walensee, and I like to make the most of each one." More than one visiting rider will long remember arriving at a lake for lunch to drop a bike on the grass and then run into the clear water for a swim with jersey and shorts still on. Bring a quick-dry towel!

The route's most challenging climb is just down the road: Brünig Pass. "The Brünig is very steep—400 meters in just 3 miles (5 km)—and the first part of the Route 9 bike path is gravel. But the views of the surrounding mountains are stunning, and there's a long coast down. You'll cover a lot of road in the afternoon, but it's flat. Eventually you'll reach Lucerne, Switzerland's most popular tourist destination. The city is beautifully preserved. Though not a large one, it seems metropolitan after the many small towns you've ridden through." More crystalline lakes and bold climbs await. You'll ride past Einsiedeln Abbey, which attracts many Catholic pilgrims, en route to Rapperswil, with its quaint medieval center. Next, you'll follow the Walensee and then the Rhine to the Liechtenstein border before reaching the hamlet of Sax. "The ride along Lake Walensee is rather surreal," John added. "You ride through a series of bike tunnels with windows that look out on the 1,500-meter cliffs that rise from the lakeshore." Your last day can be mercifully flat if you follow the Rhine to Lake Constance. Or, if you haven't had enough climbing, there's also a more mountainous route through the Appenzell region. When you reach Lake Constance, you've successfully crossed Switzerland.

JOHN KLEMME was born in Iowa, where he rode RAGBRAI. He moved to Europe more than twenty years ago and hasn't looked back. John taught English for a long time and had lots of interesting hobbies before founding Bike Switzerland and its affiliated websites. He is married, lives in Geneva and Zurich, and has a baby boy named Sasha.

If You Go

▶ **Getting There:** The ride begins in Geneva and ends near Zurich, which are both served by many international carriers.

▶ **Best Time to Visit:** May through September is high season.

▶ **Guides/Outfitters:** Several outfitters lead tours of Switzerland, including Bike Switzerland (+41 0 78 601 69 57; www.bikeswitzerland.com).

▶ **Difficulty Level:** This itinerary involves eight days of riding, with an average of 60 miles (96 km) cycling per day. It's rated moderate to difficult.

▶ **Accommodations:** My Switzerland (800-1002-0029; www.myswitzerland.com) lists lodging options in cities along the route above and throughout Switzerland.

DESTINATION

42

TAROKO GORGE

RECOMMENDED BY **Paul McKenzie**

"I had never been to Taiwan," Paul McKenzie began, "but I knew that each year it hosted a very large bicycle industry trade show—the Taipei International Cycle Show. Taiwan supplies many bicycle parts to the world market; Giant bikes, the biggest player on the planet, are made there. The equipment we make at Arkel is mostly sourced from Canada, where we're based, but a few parts are made in Taiwan. My wife, Louise, and I thought it would be good to meet some of these suppliers, so we decided to go to Taipei.

"Everywhere we travel, we look to do some cycling. However, we were not especially enthusiastic about riding in Taiwan. We knew it was a relatively small place with a large population, and crowds don't usually bode well for biking. After a little more research, we found that the interior of the island was very mountainous, and there were some roads crisscrossing the mountains. We didn't bring our bikes, figuring that if we decided to ride, we could probably rent some, as so many are fabricated there. It turns out that Giant has a great network of rental shops. You rent a bike at one shop and return it to another. You don't even have to tell the first shop where you plan to drop it off. At the show, we spoke to some local cyclists. Based on their recommendations, we decided to point ourselves in the direction of Taroko National Park and Sun Moon Lake."

Taiwan (known as the Republic of China in Beijing and other Chinese governmental circles) is roughly 100 miles east of the southeastern coast of mainland China, separated by the Taiwan Strait. Though a small landmass—245 miles long by 90 miles wide—it's the most mountainous island in the world, with more than 150 peaks topping 10,000 feet. (Taiwan's tallest peak, Jade Mountain, is 12,966 feet.) The mountains that run predominantly north to south (known as the Central Mountain Range) keep the island's twenty-three million citizens concentrated in the coastal areas. This opens up the inland to great biking possibilities. "We rented bikes on the east side of the island at the city of Hualien, and headed into the mountains," Paul continued. "The whole inside of the island, with its impressive mountain roads, was a pure dream to ride—that is, if you are up for a lot of climbing! Earthquakes and typhoons are not uncommon here, and the roads get washed out frequently. But the road that goes through Taroko National Park (Central Cross Island Highway) is closely monitored and consistently repaired."

Taroko National Park comprises 227,336 acres in northeastern Taiwan. Mountains taller than 6,500 feet cover half the park area; there are twenty-seven that top 9,800 feet. The showcase of the park is its namesake gorge, carved by the Liwu River. Fortunately for cyclists, the highway follows the gorge through the park. "The Taroko Gorge is considered one of the Asian Wonders of the World," Paul said. "It's carved very deep into the marble strata; in some places the walls are hundreds of meters high. The construction of a road along this gorge is an amazing engineering feat. The asphalt is smooth, the views of the mountains are breathtaking, there are beautiful temples along the way and even hot springs—and very few westerners in sight, let alone western cyclists!"

From Taroko, Paul and Louise continued west to the Alishan National Scenic Area, one of Taiwan's most popular tourist attractions. (Many come to hike or take a train up to the top of one mountain [Jhushan] at dawn to watch the sun rise over Yushan, East Asia's tallest mountain at 3,952 meters or 12,966 feet.) After the road topped out at an elevation of 10,745 feet, they dropped down to another of Taiwan's national treasures, Sun Moon Lake. "The clear waters and alpine setting reminded me a bit of Lake Wakatipu in New Zealand," Paul continued. "It's quite a tourist destination, attracting many Chinese visitors from the mainland. There were quite a few newlyweds there when we visited. I've never seen such a mesmerizing building as the Xiangshan Visitor Center, a remarkable modernist design. The Taiwanese have the resources to create standout structures. From Sun Moon Lake, we rode south back to civilization in the bustling city of Tainan. Here, we dropped our bikes off and took the high-speed train back to Taipei.

"Though the scenery of our ride—on par with anywhere I've been—was certainly the high point of the trip," Paul concluded, "there were other aspects of Taiwan that I appreciated. First, I felt very safe at all times. Taiwan is a wealthy country; people aren't interested in going after your stuff. When I'm biking in a place that has crime, the sense of danger takes away a lot of the fun. In Taiwan, your personal safety is better protected than anywhere in North America. I found the lodging to be quite adequate—there aren't abundant options, but they're spaced so you can ride easily from one to the next. The food is also good, especially if you enjoy seafood, though there are some odd dishes that most westerners will not have seen before. All the ingredients are there for great bike touring.

"The last thing that impressed me was the friendliness and courtesy of the Taiwanese people. Car drivers care for cyclists. Even on the mountain roads, they'll pass carefully, or let you pass. The Taiwanese are very active, very hardworking. Even teenagers seem absorbed by their work. But despite this focus, people will go out of their way to help you. As a visitor, you feel that you're in a place where things are moving so fast, growing so fast, that the country will soon be overtaking the world."

PAUL MCKENZIE is the owner of Arkel (www.arkel-od.com), a manufacturer of high-quality panniers. Before becoming involved in the cycling industry, Paul worked in banking and established his own construction business. An avid cyclist, Paul (along with his wife, Louise) has bike-toured the world, cycling self-supported through New Zealand, Cambodia, Vietnam, Morocco, Cuba, Chile, and Argentina, as well as numerous times in France, Europe, the United States, and Canada. "With my role at Arkel, I can now truly say that I have combined my passion for cycling with my day job!"

If You Go

► **Getting There:** Taiwan is served by a number of international carriers (through Taipei) including China Airlines (800-227-5118; www.china-airlines.com).

► **Best Time to Visit:** September to November has the most consistent weather.

► **Guides/Outfitters:** Giant has bike rental locations all around Taiwan. Several companies lead tours in Taiwan, including Grasshopper Adventures (818-921-7101; http://grasshopperadventures.com).

► **Level of Difficulty:** You'll want to allow five days to replicate the ride above. It's rated moderate.

► **Accommodations:** The Taroko National Park website (www.taroko.gov.tw) lists accommodations in the park. The Alishan National Scenic Area and the Sun Moon Lake Scenic Area websites (www.ali-nsa.net and www.sunmoonlake.gov.tw, respectively) highlight lodging options at these venues.

HILL COUNTRY

RECOMMENDED BY **Steve Coyle** & **Tammy Schurr**

"I've ridden all over the United States," Steve Coyle declared, "but I'm always happy to come back to Austin and the Hill Country. It's because of the high-quality, lightly traveled roads. As you may know, Texas has generated a lot of oil revenue over the years. Past budget surpluses have resulted in many lesser-known county roads getting paved. It's like having your own bike trails to ride on—there are very few cars, just the local farmers and ranchers. When I'm out riding, I'm likely to see one or two vehicles every thirty minutes. Some people imagine that all of Texas is flat, but that's not the case west of Austin and San Antonio. It's quite a rolling place, thanks to the limestone strata that've been worn away over the eons. There aren't huge ups and downs—it's Texas *Hill* Country, not *mountain* country, after all. But there are lots of 100- to 200-foot elevation climbs. I always enjoy cresting the next hill for that next vista. When you crest the right hill, you can get views that take your breath away."

"The network of farm-to-market roads in the Hill Country is just endless," Tammy Schurr added. "You can take a thousand wrong turns out there and not get too lost. There are many places to explore, and this makes it a really fun place to ride. Each little town seems to have its own claim to fame—a café, a museum, a brewery, a dance hall. I love the fact that there are so many gorgeous rivers—the Guadalupe, the Blanco, the Llano. They are very clear [most ultimately flow from the Edwards Aquifer], and we're constantly crossing back and forth over them. It's dry country, but thanks to all that flowing water, it's greener than you'd expect."

The Hill Country can be roughly defined as the region stretching 100 miles west from the cities of Austin (in the north) and San Antonio (in the south). The ride Tammy and Steve helped create begins in Austin, considered by some to be America's best city

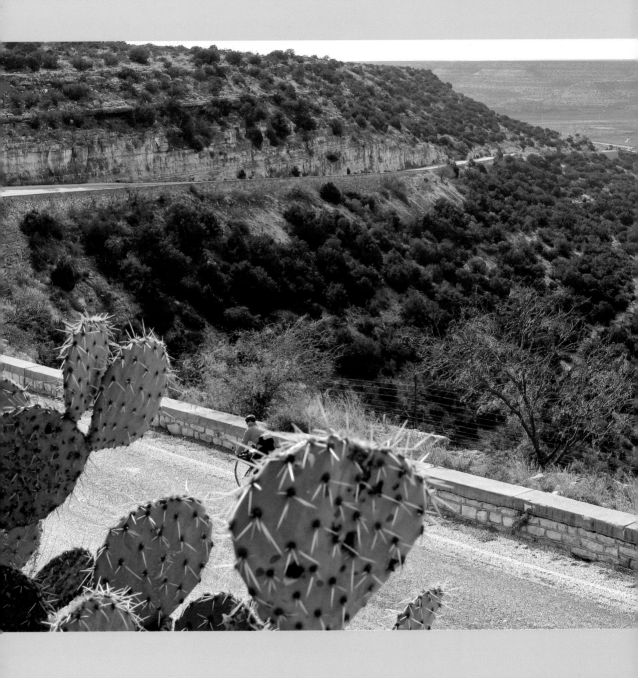

for live music. There certainly are many clubs on Sixth Street, and any serious pop music fans will want to linger a day or two in the Texas capital. But more music awaits down the road to the south in New Braunfels. This is the home of Gruene Hall, the oldest continually running dance hall in Texas and the launching point for some of the Lone Star State's more beloved acts—including George Strait, Lyle Lovett, Robert Earl Keen, and the Fabulous Thunderbirds. There's no guarantee that you'll have a brush with stardom, but you can be assured that a cold, brewed-in-Texas Shiner Bock beer will be waiting for you at Gruene Hall. The Guadalupe River flows through New Braunfels, and Steve enjoys the River Road on a Sunday morning when the water isn't crowded with tubers. "The river's lined with cypress trees, and the water is crystal clear, with some rapids, some still sections. There are many crossings on the route, and the sky and the trees reflect off the water."

It keeps getting better. The ride to the town of Blanco is considered one of the loveliest in the region. "I love riding along the Blanco River," Tammy continued. "You cross it a number of times, and it's nice to cool off your feet." "There's a little side trip you can take on the road to Blanco," Steve added, "that brings you to the Devil's Backbone. From the top of this rocky hill, you have one of the best views of the Hill Country; you can see the entire Blanco River valley." From Blanco, you continue west to Fredericksburg, a German enclave that's very popular with visitors from Texas and beyond. "Galveston was a major port in the late 1800s, and many European immigrants came into the United States through Texas," Steve explained. "That changed when the hurricane of 1900 wiped Galveston out. Many of the German immigrants found their way to Fredericksburg; when everything is green in the spring, you can see why they might have found it appealing." "Fredericksburg has a lovely downtown shopping area and a number of authentic German restaurants—and, of course, beer gardens," Tammy added. "We generally have a layover day in Fredericksburg, and there's an optional ride to a place called Enchanted Rock."

"The trip to Enchanted Rock is easily in the top five rides I've ever done," Steve continued. "There's no one out there; the road is so lightly traveled, grass is growing at the edge of the pavement! The road is wide enough for a cyclist and one car—if you see a car. The few drivers I've encountered are very courteous and will drive off on the shoulder to give you room.

"As you're approaching, you first see this big pink mound from a hilltop above the valley. It looks like nothing else around, and you can understand why the Native

OPPOSITE:
Quiet roads and
open vistas await
in the Texas
Hill Country.

DESTINATION

44

Americans were superstitious about it and wouldn't go near the rock. You soar down a hill into the state park. Enchanted Rock is one of the largest granite batholiths in the country (it covers a full square mile and rises 425 feet above the surrounding terrain). I encourage people to take some hiking shoes so they can walk to the top for a 360-degree view of the Hill Country. If there's been any rain, there are little ponds in the granite, and there are small fish in them. I don't know how they survive the dry periods." Rain also brings out the wildflowers in the surrounding countryside, especially bluebonnets. They can grow so thick that they resemble small lakes.

From Fredericksburg, you begin to push east to Austin, via Johnson City. En route, you'll pass through little Luckenbach. There's not much there beyond the one commercial building that serves as a post office/general store/bar, but country music fans will know it as a haunt for singer/songwriter Jerry Jeff Walker and as the subject of a song by Willie Nelson and Waylon Jennings. (The song's authors, reportedly, had never been to Luckenbach when they wrote the song, but they have since played there.) The Johnson City area is the sometime-home of the Hill Country's best-known cyclist, and most visitors riding through hope to catch a glimpse of Mr. Armstrong. Steve has been lucky enough to have once sighted the seven-time Tour de France winner. "I was riding with a group of friends near his ranch," he recalled. "Suddenly, there was Lance going the other way, with his then girlfriend, Sheryl Crow. 'Did you see who just rode past?' I asked my friends. By the time they turned around to look, they were almost out of sight."

STEVE COYLE is past president of the Austin Cycling Association. He helped route and has staffed Adventure Cycling Association's Texas Hill Country tour, and is also known in local circles for instigating bike trips throughout Texas and beyond. He has pedaled his bikes from Washington to Virginia and many states in between. He has a passion for bike travel that extends to his "real" job, where he is a systems analyst with Allscripts, as he commutes by bike as often as possible.

TAMMY SCHURR lives in Las Cruces, New Mexico, and has been leading and directing tours for Adventure Cycling (www.adventurecycling.org) since 2003, including trips in Arizona, Colorado, Idaho, and Texas. She's taught Smart Cycling Motorist Education at Las Cruces High's driver's ed classes, and Traffic Skills 101 and Bicycling 123 Instructor classes around New Mexico. Tammy also previously served as bicycle education coordinator for Bicycle Coalition of New Mexico. She most recently became an LCI coach for the League of American Bicyclists (www.bikeleague.org), mentoring new league cycling instructors. She's been on Adventure Cycling's Leadership Development Team and occasionally serves as a leadership training adviser during Adventure Cycling leadership training courses. Tammy can often be found researching an area she wants to ride/lead a tour, educating others about vehicular cycling, dreaming about hitting the open road, or riding her bike. Tammy says, "It is a joy to combine my passion for cycling with my vocation."

If You Go

▶ **Getting There:** The Texas Hill Country can be easily reached from either Austin or San Antonio, which are both served by many major carriers.

▶ **Best Time to Visit:** Spring and fall generally offer blues skies and moderate temperatures.

▶ **Guides/Outfitters:** Adventure Cycling Association (800-755-2453; www.adventure cycling.org) leads trips in the Texas Hill Country. The Austin Cycling Association (www .austincycling.org) offers helpful information for do-it-yourselfers.

▶ **Level of Difficulty:** This trip entails five days of cycling with an average of 60 miles (97 km) a day. It's rated moderate.

▶ **Accommodations:** The Texas state tourism website (www.traveltex.com) lists lodging options in the Hill Country. The Austin Convention and Visitors Bureau (866-645-0605; www.austintexas.org) outlines lodging options in America's live music capital.

DESTINATION

44

THE GOLDEN TRIANGLE

RECOMMENDED BY **Struan Robertson**

"Northern Thailand—the region sometimes called the Golden Triangle—is a place where you can combine a fascinating cultural tour with a variety of riding experiences," Struan Robertson explained. "In the Golden Triangle, you have the influences of all the surrounding countries coming together—Burma (Myanmar), Laos, and China. Cycling through the region, you're exposed to daily life in rural villages—such a different routine from what most visitors are used to. Many of these people spend most of their lives in relative poverty, yet they are very friendly and happy to meet foreigners—if quizzical about why you're biking, when there's a support van behind that you could ride in! We might stop by a school to rest in some shade. If the children are playing volleyball, you'll probably end up participating in a game. If we happen to ride by a wedding, we'll be invited to join in. And if you join the wedding party, you'll be expected to partake of a few drinks of *lao kao*, a home-brewed rice whiskey. It's quite potent. After a few shots of *lao kao*, your hosts will tie a string around your wrist, a sign of friendship. The rural people are always up for a good time, and most visitors enjoy this interaction. It can be hard trying to get the guests back on their bikes.

"From a riding perspective, there's great diversity. Some days you're on trails along rivers in the jungle, passing people in tribal dress. Other times you're on tarmac, climbing over a mountain pass. The first half of the trip is mostly in the jungle areas, the latter more in the mountains. The area is very populous and there's a sense of constant activity, yet there's not much traffic, especially on the secondary roads. It's a mountainous region, and there aren't many flat rides, but most of the big climbs are optional. Along the way, there are ancient temples, expansive rice paddies, and elephants. I don't think anyone will be bored by the riding!"

The Golden Triangle (which takes in mountainous regions of adjoining Burma and Laos as well as Vietnam) is perhaps best known as a place where opium is grown and harvested for use in illicit drugs, especially heroin. In the last decade, Afghanistan has supplanted the region as the world's most prolific opium poppy producer, and Thailand has appropriated the "Golden Triangle" brand to attract tourists to the country's northern territory. These efforts seem to have been successful; the airport at Chiang Mai, the region's gateway city, reports some two million visitors a year.

Struan begins his bicycle exploration of northern Thailand in Chiang Mai and slowly makes his way north through the limestone mountains around Chiang Do and on to the very northern tip of the nation, the village of Sop Ruak, and then heads back to Chiang Mai. He shared some of the ten-day excursion's most memorable moments.

"On the third day, we start from the caves at Doi Chiang Dao, which extend deep into the mountain, which is one of Thailand's highest. The ride takes us through rice fields and up along the edge of the mountain before detouring to dirt tracks. These roads have been cut by local hill tribes—the Akha, Lisu, Lahu, and Palaung people. These people initially migrated from China and Tibet, and have their own languages and cultures. The Palaung are the most recent arrivals, and we'll often see Palaung women adorned with brass waistbands working the fields. The next day is the flattest day of the trip, taking you through the fruit and vegetable plantations of the Fang Valley. Thailand's king, Bhumibol Adulyadej, has been trying to encourage farmers to grow fruit and vegetables instead of opium. In the town of Fang, there's a restaurant I always stop at. There's a dish they serve, *khao soi*—a curry soup with noodles and either chicken or beef. It's a northern Thai specialty, and as this day is one of our longer rides, people usually enjoy two bowls. The next day is lighter in the saddle, though there's no shortage of adventure. There's a short ride to a riverside town, then we load our bikes in a longtail boat and motor downriver. Upon reaching land, there's a short ride of roughly 12 miles (20 km) to the town of Ban Ruamitr, where we swap bikes for elephants and ride up the mountain to a remote Lahu village. Here, you'll stay with a family for the night in a traditional longhouse, and you'll get a sense of rural Thai life—no electricity or running water, but ample fresh food and good company.

"The eighth day brings you to the tip of Thailand and the border with Burma and Laos; it's the longest of the tour, but it's also one of the most spectacular. After rolling through some lychee orchards along dirt paths, we return to tarmac and climb Doi Tung (Flag

Mountain). The road passes through thick forests and Shan, Akha, and Lahu tribal villages. Doi Tung is not the tallest mountain in the region, but rises sharply; as you climb, the views become more and more expansive—you can see well into Burma. Near the top there's a thousand-year-old temple—Wat Phra That Doi Tung—that's an important Buddhist pilgrimage spot. It's believed that the Buddha's clavicle resides in the temple. The mountaintop is also home to the royal villa of the princess mother, Srinagarindra, who championed the cause of the Hill tribes. After lunch on the mountaintop, there's a terrific descent down to the town of Mae Sai. It's quite steep, but on tarmac, and the vistas are fantastic. The last few miles are along the Sai River. It's a long day, but it all is worthwhile as you sit by the river in Sop Ruak, open a cold Thai beer, and look out where the two great rivers join—at the tip of the Golden Triangle."

STRUAN ROBERTSON is general manager of SpiceRoads Bike Tours, which offers high-quality, educational, and adventure-filled itineraries that highlight and focus on the diversity of landscapes found in Asia and on its people.

If You Go

▶ **Getting There:** Rides begin and end in Chiang Mai, which is served by a number of carriers, including Singapore Airlines (800-742-3333; www.singaporeair.com).

▶ **Best Time to Visit:** Northern Thailand has a tropical climate. The rainy season is from July through September; you'll likely find good conditions the rest of the year.

▶ **Guides/Outfitters:** SpiceRoads (+66 2 712 5305; www.spiceroads.com) leads trips around northern Thailand and elsewhere in Asia.

▶ **Level of Difficulty:** This tour entails nine riding days. Distances are not long, but there's some single-track riding. It's rated difficult.

▶ **Accommodations:** In Chiang Mai, Imperial Mae Ping Hotel (+66 53 283 900; www.imperialhotels.com); in Chiang Dao, Royal Ping Resort (+66 81 9802525; www.royalping.com); in Chaiprakarn, Saimoonburi Resort (www.saimoonburi.com); in Mae Salak, Huai Khum Resort (+66 5371 7438; www.huaikhum.com); in Mae Salong, Mae Salong Villa (+66 5376 5114); in Sop Ruak, Phu Chaisai Resort (+66 22602646; www.phu-chaisai.com).

WHITE RIM TRAIL

RECOMMENDED BY **Kirstin Peterson**

"I first came down to the Moab area in 1989," Kirstin Peterson started. "Friends of mine had been coming for years to ride the White Rim Trail in Canyonlands National Park. They spoke of it as a magical, legendary place. I have to admit that on my first trip to Moab, everything looked somewhat the same. I found it difficult to create landmarks for myself in this terrain. I came back the next year and took a job as a mountain bike guide—with the White Rim Trail as my first tour. As I got to know the region a bit more, I began to realize how unique this landscape is. It's so different, it's like you've gone to another world. When you can take it in from a bike, it's an even more special experience."

Canyonlands National Park encompasses 525 square miles in southeastern Utah, southwest of the outdoor recreation hub of Moab. The park preserves a pristine area of the Colorado Plateau, a remarkable patchwork of canyons, mesas, and deep river gorges eroded over the ages by the Colorado and Green Rivers and their tributaries. The Colorado, coming from the northeast, and the Green, flowing from the north, meet near the center of the park; the Cataract Canyon section of the Colorado, beloved by white-water rafters, rests just below the rivers' confluence. The park's high desert environs range from 3,700 to 7,200 feet in elevation. To the uninformed eye, it can seem nearly lifeless, though many creatures (from kangaroo rats to mountain lions) call this canyon country home, limiting their movements to dawn, dusk, and night. The rivers divide the park into four districts: the Island in the Sky, the Needles, the Maze, and the rivers themselves. The White Rim Trail circles the Island in the Sky, a mesa of sandstone cliffs that sits more than 1,000 feet above the surrounding terrain. The trail—which can accommodate four-wheel-drive vehicles as well as bicycles—runs 100 miles (160 km). (The "white rim" is a shelf of light-colored sandstone, a result of erosion.) Particularly strong riders can and

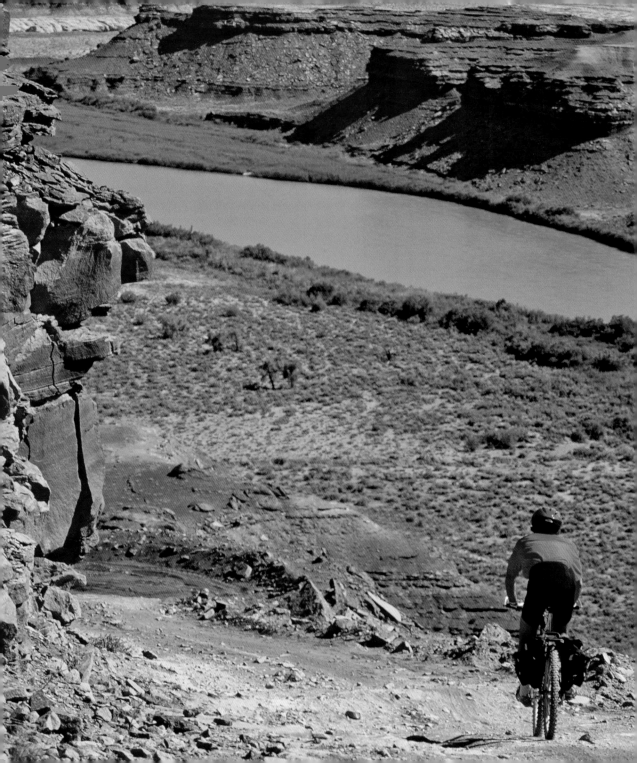

have covered the trail in one day; most will opt to complete the ride over three or four days, allowing time to enjoy the vistas and side hikes off the trail.

"The White Rim Trail appeals to a wide variety of cyclists," Kirstin continued. "There are some challenges on the way—about one good climb a day—but it's mostly moderate terrain, accessible to riders of different abilities. We stay in established backcountry campsites, where there's a pit toilet and nothing else. But a support vehicle brings all the food and camping gear, and you have everything that you need. You generally will see a few other groups out on the trail, but it's not crowded, except near the entrance on the east side." Most riders will begin the trail on that side of the park, where you drop down to the trail off "the island"—a nice descent of about 1,000 vertical feet; you'll have to gain it back at the end of the ride. Once you've reached the white rim, Canyonlands' red rock cliffs—replete with arches, towers, and myriad other formations—present themselves in all their glory. Bighorn sheep are often seen on this stretch of the ride. A few notable formations from the trail include Musselman Arch, Washer Woman Arch, and Monster Tower. If there's a climb that defines the ride, it's Murphy Hogback. "Murphy comes near the midpoint of the ride. It's a pretty stout effort for most people, about 500 feet over 2 miles (3.2 km), but feels like a lot more. Some folks will end up walking their bikes. We like to camp at Murphy, as it's the highest point on the trail beyond the start and finish. From here, you can look south toward the confluence of the Colorado and the Green Rivers. You can't quite see where the rivers come together, but you can distinguish the different characteristics of the two canyons."

Some of the highlights of the White Rim Trail come when you're not in the saddle. One noteworthy historic site a few miles off the trail is the Fort Bottom ruin, a tower-like structure above the Green River. Archaeologists believe the tower was built by Anasazi Indians in the thirteenth century, and that, like other such towers around the Southwest, it may have been used for signaling between Puebloan settlements. The same area was once used for cattle grazing, and near the river, there are remnants of a cabin built by a cowboy named Mark Walker in the late 1890s. The vistas of the river as you descend remind one of the power of the waters that formed these canyons. There are several slot canyons off the White Rim Trail, tall narrow fissures worn through the sandstone. One of the best known is the Holeman Canyon, named for a family that once grazed sheep and cattle in the Island in the Sky region. This slot canyon offers roughly 600 feet of curving, smooth-walled passageways to explore. Another unusual natural phenomenon in the park

OPPOSITE:
The Green River provides a ribbon of sustenance amid the arid majesty of Canyonlands National Park.

DESTINATION

46

is ephemeral pools or potholes. Potholes are naturally occurring basins that collect rainwater and sediment, and harbor organisms that are able to survive long periods of drought—including snails, mites, tadpoles, and fairy shrimp eggs. "If it's recently rained," Kirstin added, "the potholes come alive with critters. There are some great examples of potholes near the White Crack camping area at the southernmost point of the trail."

The expansive views from the White Rim Trail—landscapes that seem to stretch infinitely, with no sign of civilization—help define the experience. For Kirstin, the sounds of Canyonlands—or the lack of sound—also characterize the region. "At points on the ride, there are no people, no wind, no bugs, and no birds or other wildlife that make noise on a regular basis," she added. "Audio engineers have done studies and have found that Canyonlands is quieter than a professional recording studio. This amazing quiet provides a tremendous escape from most people's sense of reality."

KIRSTIN PETERSON is co-owner of Moab-based Rim Tours, which operates bike tours of Utah's canyon country, Colorado's Rocky Mountains, Arizona's Grand Canyon and Sonoran Desert, and Oregon's central Cascade Mountains. Before coming to Rim Tours, she worked as a bicycle tour guide in the California Wine Country of Napa and Sonoma.

If You Go

▶ **Getting There:** Trips begin and end in Moab, Utah. The closest commercial airports are in Grand Junction, Colorado (a two-hour drive), and Salt Lake City (four hours' drive). Salt Lake City is served by most major carriers; Grand Junction by fewer, including American Airlines (800-433-7300; www.aa.com) and United (800-864-8331; www.united.com).

▶ **Best Time to Visit:** Late March through May; September through early November.

▶ **Guides/Outfitters:** Several companies lead trips on the White Rim Trail, including Rim Tours (800-626-7335; www.rimtours.com).

▶ **Level of Difficulty:** This tour entails three or four days of riding to cover 90 miles (145 km). It's rated moderate.

▶ **Accommodations:** On the trail, you'll camp. The Moab Area Travel Council website (www.discovermoab.com) lists lodging options around Moab.

CHAMPLAIN VALLEY

RECOMMENDED BY **Gerry Slager**

White clapboarded college towns, anchored by a village green with a high-steepled church. Rolling farmlands dotted with orchards, giving way to hills and then mountains. Murmuring streams, tumbling into deep cool lakes. Vermont's Champlain Valley delivers the quintessential inland New England experience on all counts.

"Riding around the Champlain Valley, you get to see all the good things that Vermont has to offer," Gerry Slager began. "You have all the natural amenities—mountains, lakes, forests. Everything is clean; it shows the passion of the people who live here. In the little towns, there aren't billboards or fast food. But there are small local businesses, making everything from homemade chocolates and baked goods to beer and maple syrup. It's the real deal. And more often than not, when you're riding your bike on a little back road, you won't see a car."

The ride Gerry and his companions at VBT (once Vermont Bicycle Tours) have assembled explores the central section of the Champlain Valley in western Vermont. It's a low-impact tour, going light on the miles to give riders plenty of time to explore the nuances that make these intimate landscapes so special. The ride begins in Middlebury, an almost painfully picturesque college town. The Middlebury College campus, on a hill overlooking town, is a mix of stately brick buildings and modernist structures. To the west in New York State rise the craggy Adirondack Mountains, rocky and slightly imposing; to the east, the more gently rounded, tree-cloaked Greens. These views will be there for most of your trip. "One ride we like to do out of Middlebury takes us to the edge of the Green Mountains," Gerry continued. "We head south and east on back roads to Branbury State Park and Lake Dunmore, in the shade of Mount Moosalamoo. On a sunny summer day, a swim is sure refreshing." Lake Dunmore seems a set piece for idyllic memories of

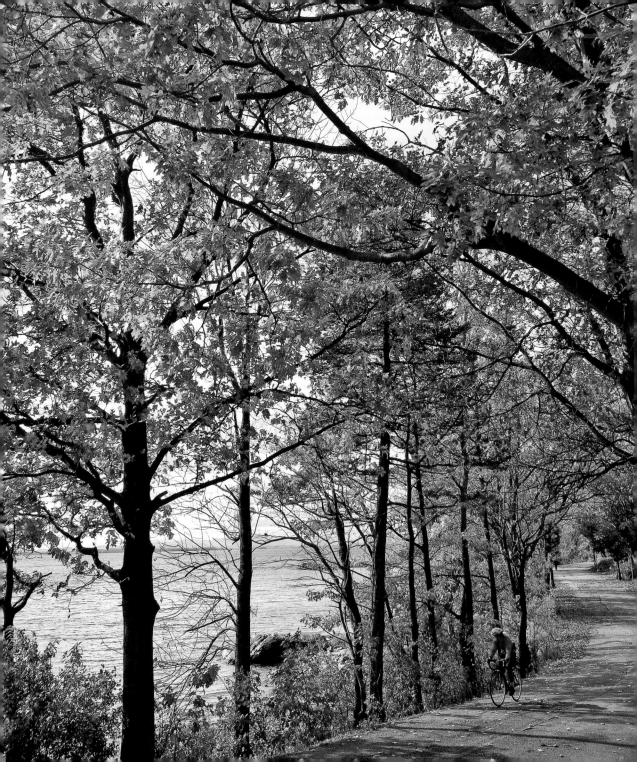

summer camps; indeed, it is the home of Camp Keewaydin, which has hosted boys since 1910 and girls (at sister Camp Songadeewin) since 1995.

OPPOSITE:
*Fall colors make
September
and October a
magical time to
tour Vermont's
Champlain
Valley.*

The following day, you'll decamp from Middlebury and make your way to the shores of Lake Champlain. En route, many of Vermont's charms, from docile dairy cows to artisan shops and mountain vistas, slowly unfold. "We roll north to New Haven Mills, past the old VBT headquarters," Gerry continued. "There's a great swimming hole there on the New Haven River with a nice sandy beach, right below the bridge. We then climb Hogback Mountain Ridge, where we'll often see Mr. Stowe, wearing his VBT hat. (He's eighty-seven as of this writing, still going strong!) From the ridge, you can look down the valley to the Bristol Cliffs and on to the Deer Leap Mountain. Soon we pass Four Hills Farm, a large dairy operation with 2,100 milking cows. [In 2010, Vermont produced more than 2.5 billion pounds of milk; some of the luckiest milk and cream is sent to the town of Waterbury, where it's converted into Ben & Jerry's ice cream and frozen yogurt.] Bristol is our lunch stop. It's a real Vermont town, not geared toward tourists, but there are great food and drink options—Bobcat Café & Brewery, Bristol Bakery, Cubbers Pizza parlor, Mountain Greens organic food market—and several craftspeople selling candles and the like. Bristol hosts the Great Bristol Outhouse Race each Fourth of July, which says something about the town's sense of humor.

"After lunch, we roll west toward Vergennes. Soon the road passes VBT headquarters, on the grounds of a former dairy farm. There's a barn facing the road where bikes are stored, and above the door there's a penny farthing bike that is made from old farm machinery. From here to Vergennes, there's a long series of fantastic rollers. Three-quarters of the way to Vergennes, there's a big oak on the left. You have to stop here and enjoy the view of Lake Champlain and the Adirondacks in the distance. Vergennes is another charming Vermont town. There's an artisan chocolatier (the Daily Chocolate), a wonderful bakery with a wood-fired oven called the Vergennes Laundry (it's in an old laundry place), a welcoming bar and grill (the Antidote), and the Black Sheep, an upscale French bistro. You may not be hungry now, but take note of the options, as you may wish to ride the 6 miles (10 km) back for dinner one of the nights you're staying out at Basin Harbor Club." Basin Harbor dates back to the turn of the last century and offers a plethora of summer activities—on the water and off—from its perch upon Lake Champlain.

Lake Champlain is a long, narrow body of water extending 110 miles (177 km) from its northernmost point just inside the province of Quebec to its southern terminus near

Whitehall, New York. Never more than 12 miles (19 km) wide, the lake forms more than half of the border between upstate New York and Vermont, and is the sixth largest lake in the Lower 48. (For not quite three weeks in 1998, Lake Champlain was America's newest Great Lake. The designation—part of an effort to secure additional federal resources engineered by Vermont senator Patrick Leahy—was quickly struck down, returning this body of water to its original status as merely a large and exceedingly scenic lake.) From Basin Harbor, you'll have a few options for exploring the lake's shoreline. "There are several loops that go south," Gerry explained, "and there's also the option to head north to Kingsland Bay State Park. This is one of my favorite rides. You'll see lots of horses, but you're lucky if one car passes." There's time for some kayaking on the lake or nearby Dead Creek Wildlife Management Area. Many visitors also enjoy the Lake Champlain Maritime Museum, which highlights the region's rich nautical history; exhibits include the schooner *Lois McClure*, a full-scale replica of an 1862-class sailing canal boat. (Thanks to its strategic location between the St. Lawrence and Hudson Rivers, Lake Champlain played a crucial role in early American history, both in the development of commerce and in the French and Indian War, Revolutionary War, and the War of 1812.)

Vermont summers are warm enough to make the water of Lake Champlain quite inviting. But for some, fall is the time to ride Vermont. "I've lived here for thirty years, and I'm still speechless when the leaves are at their peak," Gerry added. "You just pull over and stare at the mountains when they're in color. People who visit in the summer can't believe how green Vermont is. But the fall colors are unreal. It's hard to believe such colors are here."

GERRY SLAGER was living at a yoga ashram when he met a guest who told him how much she enjoyed leading VBT bicycle tours. After years of working for a steel mill in Chicago and owning a custom motorcycle shop, he returned from a driving trip that took him through ten countries to India and thought it was a great idea to try a bike tour. After thirty-three years at VBT leading hundreds of trips, he's now semiretired. Gerry has been lucky to cycle with VBT all over the United States and the world, including New Zealand, Costa Rica, Sri Lanka, Scotland, England, Holland, Canada, and Hawaii. He even met Janet Chill, his wife, at VBT!

If You Go

▶ **Getting There:** The tour described here begins and ends in Middlebury, Vermont, which is most easily reached via Burlington, where there is service from many carriers.

▶ **Best Time to Visit:** Conditions are conducive to riding June through mid-October; the latter part of the season is prime "leaf-peeping" time.

▶ **Guides/Outfitters:** Many tour companies lead rides through Champlain Valley, including VBT (800-245-3868; www.vbt.com).

▶ **Level of Difficulty:** This ride unfolds over five days, with an average 25 miles (40 km) per day. It's rated easy to moderate.

▶ **Accommodations:** VBT recommends the following riding bases: in Middlebury, Swift House Inn (866-388-9925; www.swifthouseinn.com); in Vergennes, Basin Harbor Club (800-622-4000; www.basinharbor.com).

DESTINATION

47

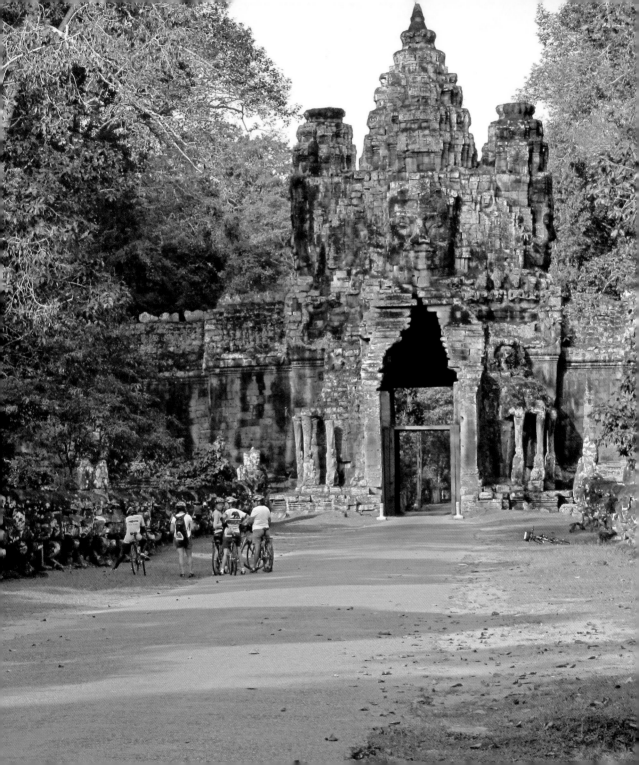

HANOI TO ANGKOR WAT

RECOMMENDED BY **Christian Chumbley**

"I always tell people who are considering a cycling trip to Vietnam that to really appreciate the adventure, you need to be as interested in Indochina as you are in riding," Christian Chumbley began. "It's first and foremost a cultural exploration. On a bike, you experience all the dynamism that is modern Vietnam. It will feel otherworldly. In Hanoi, I tell visitors, 'We're going to tell you how to cross the street.' They reply, 'What!?!' When they try to cross they understand. There's a different set of rules, a different logic operating as you try to navigate through throngs of pedestrians, cars, bicycles, and food carts.

"It's true in the countryside as well. You might be cycling past rice paddies and family mausoleums, as idyllic a setting as you could imagine. But when you come to an intersection, it's a frenetic scene that might involve water buffalo. The serenity complements the craziness, and it's all part of the experience. Being on a bike slows things down enough so you can begin to understand the logic of the place. By being on a bike, you're able to speak to children who are walking to school or chat with farmers working the field by hand (with aforementioned buffalo). Some guests look at the mileage and think '50 or 60 kilometers (31 to 37 miles)? That's not enough for me.' After the intensity of the first day, those same guests are thinking 'Maybe 60 kilometers is too much!'"

In Hanoi—which, with its tree-lined boulevards and French colonial architecture, has been dubbed the "Paris of the Orient"—you may prefer to stay on foot. The pace can be dizzying, as can the juxtaposition of old and new, as fleets of motorbikes weighed down with parcels speed past tenth-century pagodas. "One of the guides we work with—Dragon—is emblematic of current-day Vietnam," Christian continued. "His family has been in Hanoi for hundreds of years, and he's well-versed in the country's traditions. Yet he's extremely entrepreneurial. He has one foot in old Vietnam, one in the new."

OPPOSITE:
The South Gate
of Angkor Wat;
bicycle visitors
can arrive at
sunrise, before
the tour buses.

DESTINATION

48

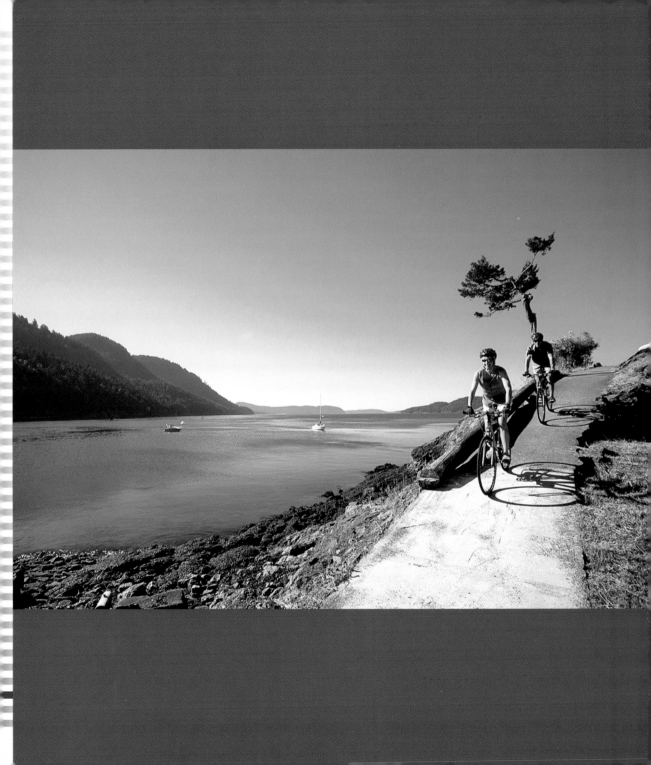

SAN JUAN ISLANDS

RECOMMENDED BY **Johannes Krieger**

"I grew up in the San Juan Islands, but didn't quite realize how special a place it is until I began running trips," Johannes Krieger explained. "Seeing the San Juans through other people's eyes made me appreciate them so much more. The islands are so close to the big metropolitan areas of Seattle and Vancouver, yet so far away from it all. The villages on each island have only local restaurants and shops and no stoplights. The scenery is tremendous and varied—there are beaches, beautiful valleys, and mountains. From a cycling perspective, there's both good climbing for advanced riders and long stretches of flatter terrain for intermediate cyclists. We don't have the mileage for the grinder who wants to do 75 or 100 miles (120 to 160 km) every day, but we do have 20- to 50-plus miles depending on which island you want to cycle. The speed limit is 35 mph on Lopez and 45 mph on Orcas and San Juan Island, so our two-lane country roads are very safe. The San Juans are best suited for those who want to stop and smell the roses, people who want to blend different activities with natural beauty and lots of wildlife. With our setting on the Strait of Juan de Fuca, we encourage visitors to go sea kayaking or whale watching so they can have a more intimate marine experience."

The San Juan Archipelago begins north of Puget Sound, roughly 60 miles (96 km) north of Seattle, and stretches nearly 100 miles (160 km). Resting between Vancouver Island and the Strait of Juan de Fuca to the west, the Strait of Georgia to the north, and the mainland of Washington to the east, the islands were the historical home of the Salish people, who traveled from island to island in cedar canoes, subsisting primarily on salmon; indeed, the inland waters are known as the Salish Sea. There are upward of seven hundred islands in the San Juan chain, though most of the area's residents live on the four largest islands—Orcas, San Juan, Lopez, and Shaw. (Some of the islands in the archi-

OPPOSITE:
Sheltered coves
and harbors are
never far away
as you tour the
San Juans.

DESTINATION

49

pelago rest in Canadian territory and are called the Gulf Islands.) The San Juans are remnants of ancient mountain ranges that geologists believe were once part of a separate continent, one that predates North America. Resting in the rain shadow of the Olympics, the climate of the islands is in stark contrast to the rest of western Washington; the San Juans see only half the rain of Seattle. The terrain—rocky bays and inlets framed by thick conifer forests—is reminiscent of the coastline of northern Maine. It's a lush, temperate landscape with enough human settlement to make provisioning easy but enough isolation to give one exposure to a unique—and mostly intact—ecosystem.

"Three of the four ferry-served islands are great for bike riding—Lopez, Orcas, and San Juan," Johannes continued. "I like to start on Lopez. It has the flattest terrain of the three, and it's a good way to get your legs warmed up, especially if you haven't been riding a lot. From the south end near Cattle Pass, there are beautiful views of the Olympic Mountains and the islands to the west. There aren't a lot of people on Lopez, and the residents are very friendly." After a ferry ride north to Orcas Island the following day, the cycling goes into higher gear—or should we say, lower gear. Here, you'll have a chance to tackle Mount Constitution in Moran State Park. "Orcas has the shape of a horseshoe with the opening facing south, and the ferry landing is on the western leg," Johannes explained. "We'll head north through Crow Valley, go around the bend in the horseshoe, and then drop down to East Sound, which is where the ascent begins—right from sea level! It's a 2,409-foot elevation gain over 8 or 9 miles (12 to 14 km). The first part has some good little inclines, but the last 2 miles (3.2 km) are pretty intense. A fair number of people end up walking their bikes. Whether you ride, walk, or hitch a ride with the support van, you must get to the top. There are 360-degree views of the Cascade Mountains on mainland Washington—on a clear day, all the way to Mount Rainier—the Olympic Mountains, even Victoria and Vancouver in British Columbia. It's considered one of the best panoramic views in the world. It's a fun descent off the mountain, and there are a number of lakes and waterfalls along the way in the park to take a dip in and cool off."

After an evening on Orcas, you'll board another ferry and head west to San Juan Island. "San Juan is the most developed of the islands," Johannes continued, "but it gives you the best blend of everything the islands have to offer. You can do a number of different things without having to travel very far. Friday Harbor is a great tourist town, with fine restaurants that use local organic food, art galleries, shops, and a rich maritime past. The kayaking is first-rate, with a good chance to come upon seals, porpoises, and orcas as you paddle along the shoreline. There's quite a bit of different terrain for riders of different abilities. There are beautiful valleys in the interior that take you past lavender and alpaca farms. Other rides hew to the coast, where you can drop your bike and head down to one of many beaches to collect shells or swim. A favorite moment comes along the west side of San Juan. There's a little climb at a spot called Bailer Hill; you then take a slight descent and another short climb, which leads you to a bend where the view suddenly opens up to Vancouver Island and the Olympic Mountain range. People just have to stop and take in how beautiful this spot is. It's not uncommon to see whales traveling along in the summer from this vantage point."

JOHANNES KRIEGER moved to San Juan Island with his parents in 1979 when he was five years old. Growing up on San Juan Island gave him a base for his love of the outdoors, kayaking, hiking, and bicycling. While attending college in 1993, Johannes founded Crystal Seas Kayaking. In 2000, Johannes, along with his wife and nephew, founded TerraTrek Bicycle and Multi-Sport Tours to offer a wider variety of activities to visitors. He now serves on the San Juan Island Parks Board and San Juan County Marine Resource Committee, and was the project manager for installing Friday Harbor's first rain garden.

If You Go

▶ **Getting There:** Ferry service is available from Anacortes (www.wsdot.wa.gov/ferries). Plane service is available on San Juan Airlines (www.sanjuanairlines.com).

▶ **Best Time to Visit:** June through September see the finest weather.

▶ **Guides/Outfitters:** A number of companies lead tours of the San Juans, including TerraTrek (888-441-2433; www.terratrek.com).

▶ **Level of Difficulty:** The tour above has four riding days, averaging 30 miles (48 km) a day. It's rated moderate.

▶ **Accommodations:** Johannes recommends the following properties: on Lopez Island, Inn at Swifts Bay (360-468-3636); on Orcas Island, Rosario Resort (360-376-2222; www rosarioresort.com); on San Juan Island, Friday Harbor House (866-722-7356; www.friday harborhouse.com).

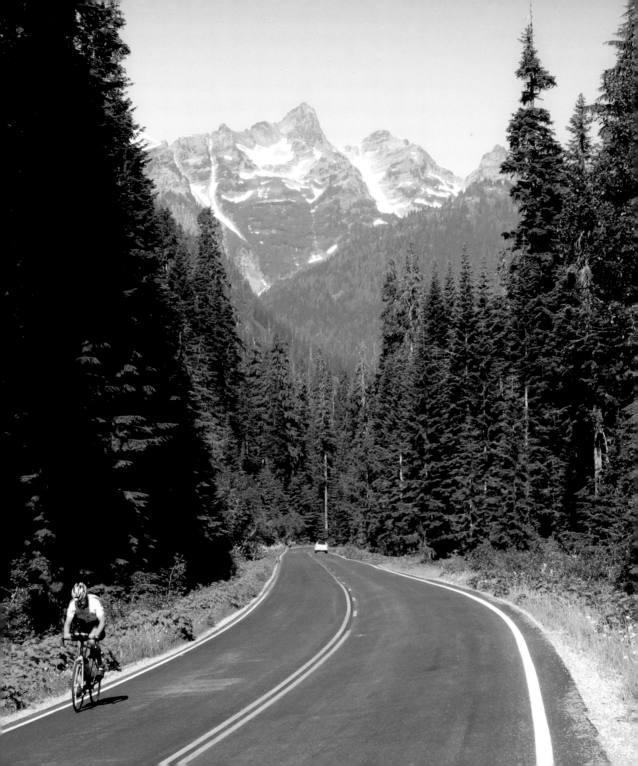

WASHINGTON STATE CHALLENGE

RECOMMENDED BY **Jan Heine**

If your idea of a great bike ride is to linger at bucolic vineyards, take in ancient ruins, and call it a day at 4 p.m. to enjoy a spa treatment, please read no further. If the idea of a casual ride of, say, 320 miles (516 km) in a twenty-four-hour period sounds appealing, do continue.

"The original idea for the Cyclos Montagnards Challenges came from reading about French constructor Paul Charrel," Jan Heine began. "Charrel lived in Lyon. During the 1930s, his goal was to ride from Lyon to the top of Mont Ventoux [in Provence] and back in twenty-four hours, a distance of 516 km (320 miles), with the final climb being unpaved and on soft gravel. Charrel tried six times, but the powerful mistral winds foiled every single one of his attempts. However, he completed other challenges, including riding from Lyon to the highest point at the foot of Mont Blanc. A few good friends of mine in Seattle—Ryan Hamilton and Mark Vande Kamp—liked the idea of a similar challenge linking our hometown with our favorite mountain destinations. We all have children now, but still like the idea of pushing boundaries, setting out on adventures, answering the question 'How far can I go?' Distance riding like this satisfies these passions. I love the simplicity of it; point A to point B and back, with a minimum of supplies and logistics. My curiosity with distance riding started in college, when I'd visit friends all over Germany. I'd ride 100, 150 miles on Saturday, spend the night, then ride back home on Sunday. Looking in our back-yard, Windy Ridge on Mount St. Helens was an obvious choice, but the distance, out and back—280 miles (450 km)—was not quite enough to fill twenty-four hours. What if we added Sunrise, the highest point of pavement on Mount Rainier? It sounded just about right at 330 hilly miles (530 km) for a full twenty-four hours. Thus, the original Cyclos Montagnards Challenge, which we dubbed the Washington Challenge, was born."

OPPOSITE: Randonneur Mark Vande Kamp cycles up Cayuse Pass (with Mount Ranier in the background) on the first running of the Washington Challenge.

The kind of challenging ride Jan and his comrades engaged upon falls under the category of *randonneuring*, a brand of long-distance cycling that was born in the 1890s. The best known of the *randonneur* routes is the Paris-Brest-Paris, a 750-mile (1,210-km) ride that began as a race but was supplanted by the Tour de France; now it's run as an endurance contest, not a race. Riders hope to complete the ride in under ninety hours. The route Jan and his comrades chose follows the western edge of Washington's Cascades, a course flanking the region's two majestic volcanic mountains, St. Helens and Rainier. On a clear day the scenery can be spectacular, but *randonneurs*—unless they're riding in far northern climes—will miss at least seven or eight hours of the sights.

"We planned our ride for around the summer solstice to have the most possible light," Jan continued. "Our total planning time was only about five hours. After dinner on June 21, 2009, the three of us met at a café in Seattle's Leschi neighborhood. After a quick cup of tea, we asked the barista on duty to sign our cards indicating our starting time—7:33 p.m. We rode past Lake Washington and into the suburbs. After briefly getting lost in an office park in Renton, we made our way into the foothills of Mount Rainier. The sun setting on Rainier was beautiful, giving us a great view of our penultimate destination. As darkness fell, we turned on our LED headlights; had they not been so bright, we might have enjoyed the stars while riding, as it was a clear night. The traffic had been light and now thinned to nothing. We reached the town of Morton by 1 a.m. and stopped for a little food and water. By 2:07 a.m., we were at Randle, the gateway to Mount St. Helens. Thirty-two miles (52 km) of uphill lay ahead.

"As we climbed, field mice scattered, and we heard owls in the trees. At the blast zone of Mount St. Helens, the hill got steeper. On one climb, I almost ran over a porcupine that was resting on the warm pavement. At 5:16 a.m., we reached Windy Ridge Overlook and looked upon Mount St. Helens's crater in the pink morning light. We had this moment to ourselves, and already felt a great sense of accomplishment. As we began our descent, to the east was the silhouette of Mount Adams. Rounding a bend, we suddenly faced Mount Rainier. Far below us were the verdant valleys reclaimed by vegetation after the tremendous volcanic blast in 1980. From here, it was mostly downhill for a time. We went into an aero tuck and reached speeds approaching 50 mph as we headed east toward the town of Packwood, where we stopped for some tea and cake. Two-thirds of our distance was behind us, and we were ahead of schedule.

"We pushed on toward Cayuse Pass, a climb that's not especially steep, but unrelenting. After a time, we reached the last part of the climb to Sunrise, a 2-mile-long ramp up the side of the ridge. As we climbed up Rainier, the wildflowers—especially the Indian paintbrush—were all in bloom. I felt like an eagle pulled high on an updraft as I looked far down on where we'd come from. There were some moments when we weren't sure we'd make it, but going downhill from Sunrise, we saw good progress, and our spirits lifted. Somewhere around the town of Enumclaw, we realized that we could reach our goal. As we hit the suburbs of Seattle, we took the Cedar River Trail to avoid the traffic. We reached the city of Renton and had an hour to cover the last 10 miles (16 km). We took care not to get lost this time around.

"When we arrived at the café where we'd started the previous evening, the same barista was working. We asked him to sign our cards. 'Didn't I see you yesterday?' he asked. 'Yes,' we said. 'You've been riding your bikes the whole time?' 'Yes,' we replied again. He gave us some cold water and congratulated us.

"It was 7:12 p.m.—we were twenty-one minutes ahead of schedule."

JAN HEINE is the editor of *Bicycle Quarterly*, a magazine about the culture, technology, and history of cycling. He has been an avid cyclist since his childhood. After racing bicycles on the road and in cyclocross for ten years, Jan now prefers *randonneuring* and long-distance riding. Apart from the Washington Challenge, his most memorable rides include four participations in Paris-Brest-Paris, as well as the Raid Pyrénéen, a 450-mile ride across the Pyrenees mountains from the Atlantic to the Mediterranean. Information about *Bicycle Quarterly* can be found at www.bikequarterly.com.

If You Go

► **Getting There:** The ride begins and ends in Seattle.
► **Best Time to Visit:** The roads on Mount St. Helens and Mount Rainier are generally open from mid-June through September.
► **Guides/Outfitters:** Jan provides details of his ride at http://cyclosmontagnards.org.
► **Level of Difficulty:** Extreme!
► **Accommodations:** The Seattle Convention and Visitors Bureau (206-461-5888; www.visitseattle.org) outlines lodging options in the greater Seattle area.

DESTINATION

50

Published in 2012 by Abrams

Text copyright © 2012 Chris Santella

Photograph credits: Title Page and Pages 2, 8, 16, 56, 80, 102, 150, 184, and 216: © Trek Travel; Pages 12, 52, 72, and 114: © VBT Bicycling and Walking Vacations; Pages 14, 24, 94, 98, 172, 196, 204, and 208: © Dennis Coello; Pages 20, 132, 146, and 212: © Backroads/David Epperson; Page 32: © Jered Gruber; Page 36: © Steve Lopushinsky; Page 42: © Dede Sullivan; Page 46: © Arlen Hall; Page 60: © Butterfield & Robinson; Page 64: © John Norris; Pages 68 and 138: © Austin-Lehman Adventures; Page 76: © Chateau de La Treye; Page 84: © Bicycle Adventures/Jill Hewins; Page 88 © Idaho Tourism; Page 106: © Enrico Pizzorni; Page 110: © Lauren Hefferon; Page 122: © Charlene Williams; Page 128: © NPS/Marc Muench; Page 154: © Nova Scotia Tourism; Page 158: © Zack Jones Photography; Page 164: Vicki Searles; Page 176: © Travel SD; Page 188: © Bike Switzerland; Page 220: © Bicycle Quarterly/Jan Heine

Library of Congress Cataloging-in-Publication Data
Santella, Chris.
Fifty places to bike before you die : biking experts share the world's
greatest destinations / Chris Santella.
p. cm.
ISBN 978-1-58479-989-4 (alk. paper)
1. Voyages and travels. I. Title.
G465.S259 2012
910.4–dc23
2012008314

Editor: Wesley Royce
Designer: Anna Christian
Production Manager: Tina Cameron
Fifty Places series design by Paul G. Wagner

This book was composed in Interstate, Scala, and Village.

Printed and bound in China
10

Abrams Image books are available at special discounts when purchased in quantity for premiums and promotions as well as fundraising or educational use. Special editions can also be created to specification. For details, contact specialsales@abramsbooks.com or the address below.

ABRAMS The Art of Books
115 West 18th Street, New York, NY 10011
abramsbooks.com